Tuberculosis Bacteriology

Tuberculosis Bacteriology: Organization and Practice

Second edition

C.H. Collins, MBE, DSc, FRCPath
Senior Visiting Research Fellow, Microbiology Department, Imperial College School of Medicine at the National Heart and Lung Institute, London, UK

J.M. Grange, MD, MSc
Director of Microbiology and Reader in Clinical Microbiology, Imperial College School of Medicine at the National Heart and Lung Institute, London, UK

M.D. Yates, BSc, MPhil
Principal Microbiologist, Mycobacterium Reference Unit, Public Health Laboratory, Dulwich Hospital, London, UK

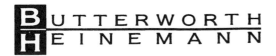

Butterworth-Heinemann
Linacre House, Jordan Hill, Oxford OX2 8DP
A division of Reed Educational and Professional Publishing Ltd

A member of the Reed Elsevier plc group

OXFORD   BOSTON   JOHANNESBURG
MELBOURNE   NEW DELHI   SINGAPORE

First published 1985
Second edition 1997

British Library Cataloguing in Publication Data
A catalogue record for this book is available from the British Library

ISBN 0 7506 2458 2

Library of Congress Cataloguing in Publication Data
A catalogue record for this book is available from the Library of Congress

Typeset by Keytec Typesetting Ltd, Bridport, Dorset
Printed and bound by Hartnolls Ltd, Bodmin, Cornwall

Contents

Preface

Throughout most of the 20th century the incidence of tuberculosis declined dramatically in the industrially developed countries but not in the developing world. The resurgence of the disease in the former countries since around 1990, the ongoing problems in other nations associated, at least in part, with the HIV/AIDS pandemic and the emergence of multidrug resistance led the World Health Organization, in 1993, to declare tuberculosis a global emergency.

The best way to prevent the spread of tuberculosis in any community is to identify the people who are excreting tubercle bacilli and to render them non-infectious to others by the provision of effective therapy. The laboratory has a central place in the diagnosis of the disease, primarily in people who are excreting large numbers of the bacilli—those who are 'smear positive'—and, secondarily, in monitoring for drug resistance, detection of people who are excreting small numbers of bacilli—those who are 'smear negative-culture positive'—and identifying other mycobacteria that might be responsible for human (and animal) disease.

In recent years, there has been increasing interest in novel diagnostic methods based on nucleic acid technology ('molecular biology'). While recognizing the importance of the development and evaluation of these new methods, the authors consider that the immediate problems of diagnosis, identification and monitoring in those countries where tuberculosis is a major public health problem are best served by techniques that are well tested and readily available. They also consider that training in these procedures should, at present, take precedence over those that are less well developed and evaluated.

C. H. Collins
J. M. Grange
M. D. Yates

Introduction: mycobacteria and mycobacterial disease

In ancient Hindu texts tuberculosis is referred to as *Rogaraj*—the king of disease, and *Rajayakshma*—the disease of kings. The first of these names, like John Bunyan's 'Captain of all of these Men of Death' emphasizes that this disease was, and in many countries still is, foremost among the causes of morbidity and mortality. The second name stresses that tuberculosis, being an infectious disease, strikes indiscriminately and affects monarch and peasant alike. Another disease of kings is leprosy, as it numbers Robert Bruce, king of Scotland, among its victims.

Both tuberculosis and leprosy are caused by members of the genus *Mycobacterium*. When originally named in 1896 in an Atlas of Bacteriology by Lehmann and Neumann, this genus contained the leprosy bacillus (*Mycobacterium leprae*) observed by Armauer Hansen in 1874 and the tubercle bacillus (*Mycobacterium tuberculosis*) observed and cultured by Robert Koch in 1882 (Koch, 1882). The name *Mycobacterium*, meaning 'fungus-bacterium', is an allusion to the characteristic fungus-like pellicle produced by the tubercle bacillus when grown on liquid media. The leprosy bacillus has never been grown convincingly *in vitro* but was included in the genus because of an important property that it shares with the tubercle bacillus—that of acid fastness. This is a characteristic staining reaction caused by the ability of mycobacteria to resist decolorization in the presence of a weak mineral acid after staining with an arylmethane dye. This staining method is described in Chapter 6.

In 1898 Theobold Smith divided Koch's tubercle bacilli into human and bovine types according to small but constant cultural differences (Smith, 1898). Later, a third mammalian type—the vole bacillus—was added by Wells (1946). These three types are often regarded as being three separate species and are named *Mycobacterium tuberculosis*, *M. bovis* and *M. microti* respectively. There is strong evidence, however, based on antigenic structure and genomic relatedness that these, together with the rather heterogeneous species *M. africanum*, are really variants of a single species. Nevertheless, in view of common usage, the separate specific names will be used in this book and the term '*M. tuberculosis* complex' will be used to refer collectively to these species.

There are two major variants of *M. tuberculosis*—the original type described by Koch, which is virulent in the guinea pig, and a more recently described variant which is attenuated in this animal. The former is found worldwide while the latter is particularly prevalent in south India and among patients of Asian ethnic origin living in other countries; accordingly, these are termed, respectively, the classical and Asian types (Collins *et al.*, 1982). The heterogeneous strains in the species *M. africanum* appear superficially to bridge the gap between *M. tuberculosis* and *M. bovis*. Those resembling *M. bovis* are found principally in West Africa (Ghana, Mauritania, Nigeria) while those resembling *M. tuberculosis* are found in more easterly African countries, notably Burundi and Rwanda. Both types, however, are found in other countries including the United Kingdom. For epidemiological purposes we divide these into two types, I and II, according to their nitratase activity (see Chapter 8), the former being negative and the latter positive. It should be stressed that this subdivision of the *M. tuberculosis* complex is purely for epidemiological purposes; the management of the patient is identical for all the above types.

In addition to the tubercle and leprosy bacilli, there are many other species of mycobacteria that live freely in the environment. These are normally harmless saprophytes but some species, as described below, are causes of human and animal disease.

The approved lists of bacterial names (Skerman *et al.*, 1980) included 41 mycobacterial species and over 20 have been published or reintroduced subsequently. The currently recognized species are listed in Table 1.1. The mycobacterial species fall into two main clusters—the slow growers and the rapid growers—which appear to have arisen as a result of a major split early in the evolution of the genus. In addition, there are a few species which are either non-

Table 1.1 The species of mycobacteria. Those included in the approved lists (Skerman *et al.*, 1980) are marked with an asterisk

M. tuberculosis complex:

*M. tuberculosis**	*M. bovis**	*M. africanum**	*M. microti**

M. avium complex (MAC) and related species:

*M. avium**	*M. intracellulare**	*M. lepraemurium**	*M. paratuberculosis**
M. sylvaticum			

Slowly growing photochromogens:

*M. asiaticum**	*M. kansasii**	*M. marinum**	*M. simiae**

Slowly growing scotochromogens:

*M. gordonae**	*M. scrofulaceum**	*M. szulgai**

Slowly growing non-chromogens:

M. branderi	*M. celatum*	*M. gastri**	*M. haemophilum**
*M. farcinogenes**	*M. malmoense**	*M. nonchromogenicum**	*M. shimoidei*
M. shinshuense	*M. triviale**	*M. terrae**	*M. ulcerans**
*M. xenopi**			

Rapid growers:

M. aichense	*M. agri*	*M. aurum**	*M. austroafricanum*
M. chelonae	*M. chitae**	*M. chubuense*	*M. diernhoferi*
*M. duvalii**	*M. fallax*	*M. flavescens**	*M. fortuitum*
*M. gadium**	*M. gilvum**	*M. komossense**	*M. neoaurum**
M. obuense	*M. parafortuitum**	*M. phlei**	*M. porcium*
M. pulveris	*M. rhodesiae*	*M. senegalense**	*M. smegmatis**
M. sphagni	*M. thermoresistibile**	*M. tokaiense*	*M. vaccae**

Non-cultivable or very poorly growing species:

*M. leprae**	*M. genavense*	*M. confluentis*	*M. interjectum*
M. intermedium			

cultivable, notably *M. leprae*, or which grow very poorly in culture media. Some of these have been isolated from cases of AIDS-related disseminated disease and characterized by sequence differences in their ribosomal RNA (see Chapter 10): they include *M. genevense*, *M. interjectum*, *M. intermedium* and *M. confluentis* (Kirschner *et al.*, 1993). The older literature contains some species names that are no longer valid; the more commonly encountered of these names and their currently valid synonyms are listed in Table 1.2.

From the purely clinical point of view, mycobacteria are divisible into three groups (Grange and Collins, 1983):

(1) The obligate pathogens—the *M. tuberculosis* complex and *M. leprae*;
(2) species that normally live freely in the environment but also cause 'opportunist' infections in humans; and
(3) species that never, or with extreme rarity, cause disease.

The species in the second group have been referred to by a number of rather unsatisfactory collective epithets including 'anonymous', 'atypical', 'tuberculoid', 'non-tuberculous' and 'mycobacteria other than tubercle' (MOTT) bacilli. In this book the term 'environmental mycobacteria' (EM), will be used. The EM differ from the obligate pathogens in several important ways. They are rarely, if ever, transmitted directly from host to host: they are almost always acquired directly from the environment. Consequently, a major factor determining the occurrence of infections caused by the various species is their distribution in the environment. This is influenced by many factors and varies considerably from region to region. As these species live freely in the environment they may occur as harmless residents of the skin, gut or upper respiratory tract of humans and animals. As a result, the isolation of such a bacillus from a clinical specimen does not *per se* imply that it is responsible for disease. There is no absolute division between groups 2 and 3 as, especially in the era of HIV infection and

Table 1.2 Synonyms

Former name	Official name
'M. aquae'	M. gordonae
'M. abscessus'*	M. chelonae
'M. balnei'	M. marinum
'M. borstelense'	M. chelonae
'M. buruli'	M. ulcerans
'M. friedmannii'	M. chelonae
'M. giae'	M. fortuitum
'M. habana'	M. simiae
'M. johnei'	M. paratuberculosis
'M. littorale'	M. xenopi
'M. luciflavum'	M. kansasii
'M. marianum'	M. scrofulaceum
'M. minetti'	M. fortuitum
'M. peregrinum'*	M. fortuitum
'M. platypoecilus'	M. marinum
'M. ranae'	M. fortuitum
'M. runyonii'	M. chelonae

*It has been proposed that *M. abscessus* and *M. peregrinum* should be re-introduced as valid species (Kusunoki and Ezaki, 1992)

iatrogenic immunosuppression, no mycobacterium can be regarded with confidence as being totally benign.

Tuberculosis

This is by far the most frequently encountered mycobacterial disease in the world. Among the infectious diseases, it is the commonest cause of death in adults and, after acute respiratory and diarrhoeal diseases, in children. It remains a major public health problem in most developing nations, in which between 0.1% and 0.3% of the population become ill each year. Although the incidence of the disease declined dramatically in the industrially developed nations during the 20th century, there has been a distinct increase in incidence in many of them since the mid-1980s. The problem has been fuelled by the HIV pandemic, increasing urban deprivation and the emergence of multidrug resistance. The worldwide threat to human health is now so serious that, in 1993, the World Health Organization (WHO) took the unprecedented step of declaring tuberculosis a global emergency. This has led to an increased awareness of the disease by physicians and the general public.

According to WHO (Kochi, 1991), about one third of the world's population has been infected by the tubercle bacillus. Each year, between 8 and 10 million cases of active tuberculosis develop from the infected pool and infect a further 100 million people. The annual mortality is around 3 million (2 million adults and 1 million children). Put another way, tuberculosis causes more than 5000 deaths every day or one about every 15 seconds. Unless radical changes in tuberculosis control are soon instituted, the incidence of the disease will continue to rise and the annual number of deaths could reach 4 million by the year 2004. At present, control programmes and supporting services, including tuberculosis laboratories, are grossly underfunded.

The impact of the HIV pandemic on tuberculosis has been, and will continue to be, a cause of great concern. Indeed, so serious is the problem that HIV and tuberculosis have been termed 'the cursed duet' (Chretien, 1990). Whereas non-immunocompromised people infected with the tubercle bacillus have a 10% chance of developing overt tuberculosis some time during the remainder of their lives, the risk rises to 50% in HIV-positive individuals during their shortened lifespan, with an annual chance of developing overt disease of 8-10%. The interval between infection and disease is often only a few months and this, together with the high chance of developing disease, has led to a number of serious outbreaks which have been particularly well documented in New York (Rieder, 1994). In 1995 around 8% of all cases of tuberculosis worldwide, and 20% in sub-Saharan Africa, were HIV-related and predictions for future trends in Africa and elsewhere are very worrying. Although tuberculosis in HIV-positive people responds to chemotherapy (unless there is a problem of drug resistance) the mortality over the following two years is high, possibly because of a synergy between the immunosuppressive properties of the two pathogens.

Multidrug resistance has emerged as a serious threat to tuberculosis control in many developed and developing nations. By definition, a multidrug-resistant strain is one that is resistant to the two principal drugs used in modern short-course chemotherapy—rifampicin and isoniazid—with or without additional resistances. Such resistance renders standard short course regimens ineffective and treatment for longer durations with less effective but more toxic and expensive drugs is required. Even under the best medical conditions, the prognosis is poor. In New York where new drugs are available and treatment is supervised, death occurred within two years of diagnosis in about 45% of patients, rising to 85% in those who are HIV positive. Multidrug resistance has arisen as a result of poor organization and supervision of antituberculosis chemotherapy and WHO (1995) now advises that all drugs should be administered under direct supervision—the so-called directly observed therapy, short course regimen (DOTS). HIV infection does not appear to cause drug resistance *per se* but it greatly accelerates its spread in susceptible communities. Many such outbreaks have been described, principally in the USA, but also in France, Spain, Italy and the United Kingdom.

The lung is the most frequently infected organ in tuberculosis but other sites in which the disease often occurs include lymph nodes, bone, kidneys, the reproductive system, intestine, skin and central nervous system. No organ or structure, however, is exempt from infection and occurrence of disease in unusual sites may pose serious diagnostic problems. Tuberculosis patients who are HIV positive, notably those with CD4+ counts of under $50 \times 10^6/l$, often present with atypical forms of tuberculosis, notably pulmonary infiltrations with little or no cavity formation, non-symmetrical lymphadenopathy and/or widely disseminated disease.

Tuberculosis is usually acquired by the inhalation of small moist cough droplets, about 5 μm across, containing a few bacilli. Such particles lodge in a peripheral part of the lung. The events following such infections vary enormously from patient to patient but it is, nevertheless, possible to discern a general pattern of progression or 'timetable' of disease (Wallgren, 1948). Local multiplication of bacilli at the site of implantation leads to the formation of a small lesion termed the Ghon focus. Bacilli are carried by the lymphatics from this focus to the draining lymph nodes where additional bacillary multiplication occurs. The lesion consisting of the Ghon focus and the enlarged regional nodes is termed the primary complex (Figure 1.1).

The protective immune response in tuberculosis is of the 'cell-mediated' type and is due to the activation of macrophages by chemical mediators termed lymphokines released by lymphocytes following their stimulation by the appropriate antigens. Activated macrophages and lymphocytes form a compact aggregate around the bacilli, thereby creating the histological structure termed the granuloma. Such 'cell-mediated immunity' (CMI) takes about 10 days to develop and is distinct from the necrotizing 'delayed hypersensitivity' (DTH) which causes gross tissue destruction and pulmonary cavity formation. Both CMI and DTH manifest as positive skin test reactivity to tuberculin.

In about 95% of infected non-immunocompromised individuals, the primary complex heals while in the remaining 5% the disease process may progress in one or more ways to give rise to overt primary tuberculosis. Bacilli may spread from the primary complex to other sites by the lymphatic and blood streams, particularly in young children. This may lead to tuberculous meningitis, which often occurs about three months after infection, or to more slowly progressive lesions in bones, joints or the kidney, which are usually detected a year or more after infection. A more widespread dissemination leads to miliary tuberculosis with small granulomas resembling millet seeds (Latin: *milium*, a millet seed)

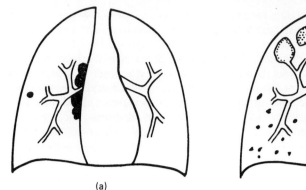

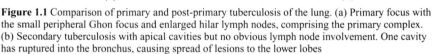

(a)   (b)

Figure 1.1 Comparison of primary and post-primary tuberculosis of the lung. (a) Primary focus with the small peripheral Ghon focus and enlarged hilar lymph nodes, comprising the primary complex. (b) Secondary tuberculosis with apical cavities but no obvious lymph node involvement. One cavity has ruptured into the bronchus, causing spread of lesions to the lower lobes

throughout the body. Alternatively, the primary focus or enlarged lymph nodes may erode into the pleural or pericardial spaces, a lymph node may erode into a bronchus causing a spreading endobronchial infection or a grossly enlarged node may compress a bronchus, causing pulmonary collapse (epituberculosis). Vaccination with Bacille Calmette-Guérin (BCG) reduces the incidence of primary tuberculosis but there is uncertainty as to its mode of action.

In people in whom the primary complex resolves, some bacilli may persist in a poorly understood dormant state for several years or even decades, eventually reactivating to cause post-primary tuberculosis in about 5% of those initially infected. Alternatively, post-primary tuberculosis may be due to exogenous reinfection. The usual site for such reactivation or reinfection is the apical region of the lung. Unlike primary disease, post-primary pulmonary tuberculosis is usually characterized by tissue necrosis and the formation of cavities which, as described below, play an important role in the transmission of the bacilli. Such cavity formation is the result of inappropriate immune reactivity and, as mentioned above, it is less evident or absent in immunocompromised patients, notably those who are HIV positive.

Not all patients with tuberculosis are infectious. For transmissibility to occur, there must be a communication between the active lesion and the outside world. Such communication usually results from the rupture of a tuberculous pulmonary cavity into a bronchus: this enables the bacilli to be expectorated in the sputum. As a rule, only patients whose sputum contains enough bacilli to be seen on a standard but competent microscopical examination are infectious. Such patients are said to have open or smear-positive disease. As a further general rule, patients with primary disease, in whom cavity formation is rare, tend not to be infectious.

Leprosy

This disease is considered in Chapter 11.

Other human mycobacterioses

Other mycobacterial diseases of humans are, in relation to tuberculosis and leprosy, uncommon. Their incidence has, however, increased dramatically in some populations as a result of the HIV pandemic. Two environmental mycobacteria cause specific named diseases while the remainder cause less specific infections which often mimic the manifold forms of tuberculosis.

The two named diseases are Buruli ulcer—caused by *M. ulcerans* and swimming pool granuloma (also called fish tank granuloma or fish fancier's finger) caused by *M. marinum*.

Disease caused by *M. ulcerans* was first described in the Bairnsdale region of Australia. Later, '*M. buruli*' was isolated from skin ulcers in the Buruli district of Uganda and was found to be identical to *M. ulcerans*. The disease was subsequently found in several restricted localities within the tropics. Although never cultivated from the environment, it is thought to be a free-living organism that is introduced into the skin of patients by spikes on vegetation. The bacilli multiply in the subcutaneous fat which undergoes necrosis and liquefaction. Eventually the overlying skin breaks down and the necrotic fat is discharged leaving a deeply undermined ulcer. At this stage numerous bacilli are present at the advancing edge of the lesion and, as in lepromatous leprosy, the specific immunological reactivity is suppressed. Almost all patients reach a point when, for unknown reasons, immune reactivity appears, bacilli disappear and healing commences. Unfortunately, fibrosis and contractures occurring during healing usually leave the patient with a severe disability or disfigurement. For a review of Buruli ulcer and its treatment see Meyers (1995).

Mycobacterium marinum occurs in swimming pools and fish tanks and enters the skin through abrasions acquired by swimmers or fish fanciers. The infection usually manifests itself as a raised, pink, soft, warty lesion and in some cases one or more secondary and proximal lesions develop along the route of the draining lymphatics, a condition termed sporotrichoid spread as it is seen in the fungal infection sporotrichosis. The disease is usually benign and self-limiting: more serious infections involving tendons and joints have been reported but these are extremely rare. For further clinical details see Collins *et al.* (1985).

The other mycobacterial species that infect humans cause much less characteristic lesions. The relative incidence of the species involved varies from region to region and is related to the occurrence of the species in the environment. The most frequently encountered slowly growing species are *M. avium* and the closely related *M. intracellulare*. Indeed many bacteriologists refer to them as the *M. avium* complex (MAC) or, less often, as *M. avium-intracellulare* (MAI), while others, especially workers in the USA, add the distinct species *M. scrofulaceum* and call the resulting cluster the MAIS complex. Also closely related to *M. avium* are three pathogens of animals, namely, *M. paratuberculosis*, the cause of hypertrophic enteritis or Johne's disease of cattle; *M. lepraemurium*, the cause of a disease superficially resembling leprosy in rodents and cats; and *M. sylvaticum*, a species resembling both *M. avium* and *M. paratuberculosis* and causing disease in wood pigeons. Other frequently encountered slowly growing species are *M. kansasii*, *M. scrofulaceum* and *M. xenopi*. Less frequent as causes of disease among the slow growers are *M. branderi*, *M. celatum*, *M. genevense*, *M. haemophilum*, *M. malmoense*, *M. simiae* and *M.*

szulgai. There are only two rapidly growing species of importance as pathogens: *M. chelonae* (previously *M. chelonei*) and *M. fortuitum*. Other species are not regularly encountered as pathogens but, especially in this age of the HIV pandemic and of iatrogenic immunosuppression, any mycobacterium must be regarded as a potential cause of disease until proved otherwise. There are a few reports of diseases due to *M. flavescens*, *M. gordonae*, *M. triviale* and *M. nonchromogenicum*. For a list of pathogenic mycobacteria according to the diseases they cause in humans and animals, see Table 8.1 (p. 70).

There are four main classes of disease caused by environmental mycobacteria, in addition to the named diseases, Buruli ulcer and swimming pool granuloma, described above.

1.   Lymphadenopathy.   This usually involves the cervical nodes and is caused by the *M. avium* complex in 80–90% of cases. The disease is almost always unilateral and most cases occur in young children. In the absence of an immuno-suppressive disorder such infections are mostly self-limiting, particularly if the nodes are totally excised, as is often done for diagnostic purposes. The incidence of this mycobacteriosis is reduced by neonatal BCG vaccination.

2.   Progressive lung disease.   Most cases are in elderly people, usually male, with underlying lung damage, though younger patients with no apparent predis-posing factor are occasionally affected. This disease often resolves on appro-priate chemotherapy (Chapter 9). A minority of cases fail to respond to chemotherapy, and surgery is indicated if the disease is localized and there is adequate pulmonary function. The usual causes are the *M. avium* complex, *M. kansasii*, *M. malmoense*, *M. scrofulaceum* and *M. xenopi* but cases caused by several of the other species listed above have also been reported.

3.   Inoculation mycobacterioses.   Lesions result from the implantation of mycobacteria into tissues by injections, accidental trauma and surgery (Grange *et al.*, 1988). A number of cases of 'sterile' post-injection abscess have been shown to be caused by the rapid growers *M. fortuitum* and *M. chelonae*. Such infections are usually self-limiting or respond to adequate curettage and drainage but the same species have caused a number of widespread and life-threatening infections following major surgery, particularly open-heart surgery (Grange, 1992). These species have also caused several cases of keratitis which, particularly when caused by *M. chelonae*, respond poorly to chemotherapy and usually require corneal transplantation (Khooshabeh *et al.*, 1994). Very occa-sionally, superficial skin infections mimic lupus vulgaris or swimming pool granuloma.

4.   Disseminated disease.   Involvement of many organs may occur in those who are immunosuppressed, particularly children with congenital defects in cell-mediated immunity, people with hairy cell leukaemia and certain other neoplasias and transplant recipients. In recent years such disease, usually caused by the *M. avium* complex, has emerged as one of the commonest complications of AIDS. In the USA, this disease occurs in over 30% of such patients, almost always after the appearance of other AIDS-defining disorders. It is also common in Europe but not in Africa, despite the occurrence of members of the *M. avium* complex in the African environment. The bacilli are found in large numbers in the blood, bone marrow and other organs. The intestinal wall is often infiltrated and the bacilli are found in the faeces. It is not clear whether the disease is the result of reactivation of latent infection acquired early in life or the result of recent direct infection from the environment. In many cases, treatment improves the quality of the remainder of the patients' lives.

It is clear therefore that the mycobacteria are the cause of a very important group of infectious diseases of humans. Despite much research since the time of Koch, attempts to develop an immunological or biochemical diagnostic test for these infections have proved unsuccessful. Accordingly a good bacteriological service is essential for the detection and diagnosis of these diseases as well as for their subsequent management.

For a more comprehensive review of mycobacterial disease see Grange (1996).

The role and scope of the tuberculosis laboratory

Laboratory services play a pivotal role in the diagnosis, management and epidemiological investigation of tuberculosis and the other mycobacterial diseases reviewed above (Salfinger and Morris, 1994). The roles of the laboratory are various and differ from region to region according to local requirements and financial constraints. These roles may be summarized as follows:

- detection of acid-fast bacilli in sputum and other specimens by microscopy;
- culture of clinical specimens for mycobacteria;
- determining whether an isolate is *M. tuberculosis* or one of the other species;
- identifying these other species;
- conducting drug susceptibility tests;
- consulting clinicians on the diagnosis and management of disease;
- collecting and analysing data for epidemiological purposes;
- teaching, including the training of technical staff;
- research and development.

Not all of these functions are carried out by every laboratory. In most countries bacteriological services are arranged in a hierarchical fashion as described in Chapter 2.

In regions with a high incidence of tuberculosis but with limited healthcare resources, the major role of the medical services is to detect infectious cases and to treat them. There is strong evidence (Rouillon *et al.*, 1976) that, for practical purposes, only those patients whose sputum contains enough bacilli to be detected by microscopy are infectious. There is little to be gained in detecting additional cases by more expensive cultural techniques unless these patients can also be offered courses of chemotherapy.

The culture of specimens for mycobacteria is much more costly than microscopy. It requires incubators, facilities and materials for preparation of media and the necessary skilled staff to undertake decontamination, inoculation of media and detection of positive cultures. Nevertheless, it serves three major purposes. Firstly, as indicated above, it detects patients whose sputum contains insufficient bacilli for them to be seen microscopically. It has been estimated that, for microscopic detection, there must be between 5000 and 10 000 acid-fast bacilli in every ml of sputum while cultural techniques will detect as few as 10 viable bacilli (Rouillon *et al.*, 1976). Secondly, culture enables a definite identification of the bacillus to be made. This is not so important in areas where tuberculosis is very common as the great majority of isolates will be *M. tuberculosis*, but in countries in which there is a very low incidence of this disease a substantial number of isolates will be of other species. Thirdly, culture is an essential prerequisite for drug susceptibility testing although, as described in Chapter 10, molecular techniques for determining drug susceptibilities without the need for prior cultivation of the bacilli are being developed.

In most parts of the world, culture of mycobacteria is based on conventional techniques that have changed little over the last half century. In some regions, more rapid, but more costly, radiometric techniques are in regular use and rapid non-radiometric methods are becoming available. Such technology permits the introduction of 'fast track' diagnostic services where there is a particular need, such as areas with a high incidence of multidrug-resistant tuberculosis (Salfinger and Pfyffer, 1994). In addition, as described in Chapter 10, nucleic acid-based technology ('molecular biology') is being applied to the rapid diagnosis and identification of mycobacteria in clinical specimens. These techniques include specific nucleic acid probes and amplification techniques (polymerase chain reaction and related methods). Considerably more developmental work is required before these techniques are able to replace the conventional ones and, if and when they do so, it is likely that they will be used principally in the form of commercially available kits.

In many respects, the role of the veterinary mycobacteriology laboratory is similar to that concerned with human disease although, as infected animals tend to be slaughtered rather than treated, drug susceptibility testing is rarely undertaken. Veterinary laboratories are concerned principally with the isolation of *M. bovis*, bird-pathogenic strains of *M. avium*, and *M. paratuberculosis*. From time to time, though, there may be a need to investigate outbreaks of mycobacterial infections caused by other species among captive or free-living animals.

In addition to the above functions, central medical and veterinary reference laboratories are often responsible for the quality of mycobacteriology practised in their country (Chapter 2, p. 22). They may also be responsible for the training of staff who work in the dependent laboratories. Reference laboratories are often also the source of both medical and technical advice and they often initiate, or participate in, basic and clinical research programmes.

Although in some countries tuberculosis is a notifiable disease, this surveillance technique is not perfect—many cases go unreported, notably non-pulmonary cases. Estimates of the incidence of the disease based on the number of positive cultures reported by laboratories are also unsatisfactory as bacilli are not cultured from all cases of the disease. Taken together, however, a fairly accurate estimation of the incidence of disease can be reached. Examination of the tubercle bacilli by using, for example, the methods for subdivision described in Chapter 8, may yield further important epidemiological information. Thus, for example, the behaviour of tuberculosis caused by *M. bovis* in the community may be studied and differences in the bacterial population between various ethnic groups of patients may be found. The recently introduced DNA fingerprinting techniques described in Chapter 10 provide very discriminative methods for investigating the transmission of disease in the community and for the study of epidemics. The results of drug susceptibility testing are also of epidemiological importance as they draw attention to breakdowns in good therapeutic practice and delineate populations in which there is a high incidence of drug resistance.

Epidemiological studies on disease caused by other mycobacterial species can be conducted only if laboratory reports are available. Such studies are of importance as they delineate populations at risk from such disease and also point to potentially dangerous sources of infection. The colonization of water-softening resins in renal dialysis machines (Azadian *et al.*, 1981) is one example. In some cases, though, 'epidemics' of such disease may be artefactual as a result of contamination of the specimens or culture media. Reference specialists, with their knowledge of the ecology of mycobacteria, may be able to detect the origin of such contamination (Collins *et al.*, 1984).

2

The tuberculosis laboratory

Grades of laboratories

State health authorities determine the level of tuberculosis laboratory services that they can afford or deem necessary. Several systems have been proposed, both in developed and developing countries, for grading laboratories according to the complexity of the service they offer. These include those of the UK Public Health Laboratory Service (1966); the Centers for Disease Control (see Richmond and McKinney, 1993); the American Thoracic Society (1983) and of Mitchison (1982). These grades fit quite well with the current system for classifying laboratories according to the hazards presented by the biological agents (World Health Organization, 1993a; Commission of the European Communities, 1990). See Table 3.1, p. 27.

These may be adapted to give three containment levels of tuberculosis laboratories:

TB level 1. These are usually single rooms or parts of another laboratory at the primary health care or local hospital level. Tuberculosis investigations are restricted to the collection and despatch of specimens to a higher level laboratory.

TB level 2. These laboratories may be in larger, e.g. district, hospitals and are part of a pathology laboratory complex. The work includes examining direct smears and, in some, culturing specimens, but the cultures are usually sent to a higher grade laboratory for incubation and further tests.

TB level 3. These more specialized laboratories examine direct smears and culture specimens for mycobacteria. Some may do no more than this and send the cultures to other TB level 3 laboratories. Others continue with the identification of the mycobacteria to species level and do antimicrobial drug susceptibility tests. The highest grade of TB level 3 laboratories usually do research and function as training centres and as reference laboratories.

Laboratory design

The TB level 1 laboratory

This is usually no more than a side room where only the most simple laboratory investigations such as blood microscopy and urine examination are carried out.

No tuberculosis bacteriology is done, but specimens may be collected for transmission to higher level laboratories.

The TB level 2 laboratory

The design and physical requirements of a TB level 2 laboratory, adapted for work with tuberculous materials from the specifications of the World Health Organization (1993a) and other organizations (see, for example, Commission of the European Communities, 1990; Richmond and McKinney, 1993) are listed in Table 2.1.

Although most regulatory bodies in developed countries insist that work with tuberculous materials is conducted in TB level 3 laboratories, this is not always practical in developing countries. Given good staff training and supervision, it is probably safer to work at TB level 2 without a microbiological safety cabinet (see below) than in an unsafe TB level 3 room where the cabinet gives no protection, especially where the electricity supply is unreliable. It may also be argued that the staff in many of these units in developing countries are more exposed to tuberculosis outside the laboratory than when they are working in it, and that resources are better deployed on prevention and treatment of the disease in the community than on high level laboratory design.

Figure 2.1 shows how such a TB level 2 tuberculosis laboratory could be designed. If it is not possible to fit a reliable microbiological safety cabinet there should be as much natural ventilation as possible and the tuberculosis bench should be placed so that air from open windows does not blow across it and carry any infectious particles that may be released during the work into the face of the worker.

The laboratory will need an incubator, a refrigerator and, possibly, a centrifuge. An autoclave is also necessary but need not be in the same room. Hand washing facilities are essential, either within the room or just outside it.

The TB level 3 laboratory

As the work in this laboratory is likely to generate infectious aerosols, the minimum design features should be such as to protect workers from inhaling

Table 2.1 Design features for TB levels 2 and 3 laboratories

	TB level 2	TB level 3
Separate laboratory accommodation	No	Yes
Separate record accommodation	No	Yes
Access limited to authorized persons	Yes	Yes
Room sealable for disinfection	Yes	Yes
Hand wash basin	Yes	Yes
Internal observation window	Optional	Yes
Benches impervious to water, acids, solvents	Yes	Yes
Equipment shared with other laboratories	Yes	No
Air conditioning	No	Optional
Air recirculated in building	Optional	No
Negative pressure in room	No	Yes
Filtered extract air	No	Yes
Microbiological safety cabinet(s)	Optional	Yes
Safe storage of infectious materials	Yes	Yes

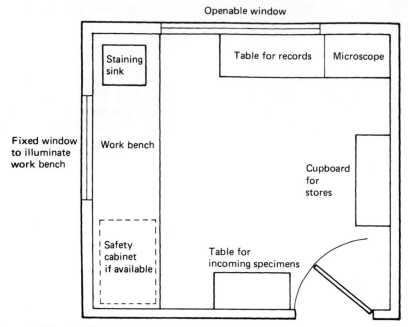

Figure 2.1 Plan for a TB level 2 laboratory

them. The physical requirements of a TB level 3 laboratory, adapted for work with tuberculous materials from the specifications of the World Health Organization (1993a) and other organizations (see, for example, Commission of the European Communities, 1990; Richmond and McKinney, 1993) are listed in Table 2.1 and discussed below.

Contrary to a common belief among health service administrators, architects and engineers, level 3 laboratories do not need sophisticated and expensive air conditioning. Indeed, many of the problems and failures of microbiological safety cabinets in new laboratories are directly attributable to such airflow and extraction systems, quite apart from the fact that incorrect pressure gradients may place workers in other rooms at risk from airborne infections. The principle of a level 3 laboratory is that during working hours air is continually extracted to the outside of the building, either through a microbiological safety cabinet or through a simple extract fan in the wall or window. A pressure gradient is thus established so that air always flows from the corridor or other laboratories to the containment laboratory and finally outside the building, thus preventing the dispersal of airborne micro-organisms to other parts of the building. As the exhaust air from safety cabinets is filtered to remove bacteria, and the dilution factor at the point of exhaust is considerable, there is a negligible risk to people in the vicinity. Figure 2.2 offers a design for a simple TB level 3 tuberculosis laboratory which is, in effect, an annex to a level 2 laboratory. The figure also shows the directions of airflows. A more sophisticated TB level 3 unit, suitable for research as well as diagnostic work, is shown in Figure 2.3.

Internal windows, either in the doors or walls, should be included in the design so that workers in the level 3 room are under surveillance in case of

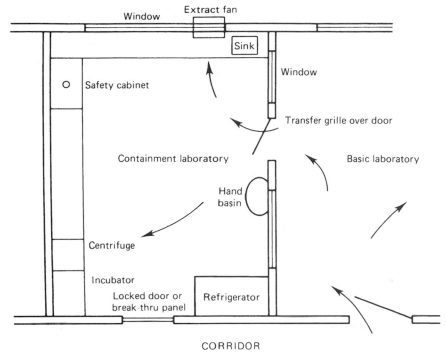

Figure 2.2 Plan for a TB level 3 laboratory. Arrows indicate direction of airflow

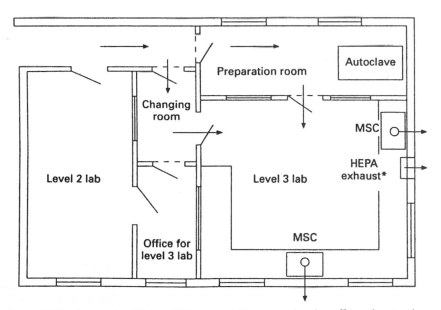

Figure 2.3 Plan for a more sophisticated laboratory, with separate changing, office and preparation rooms. Arrows indicate direction of airflow; – – –, transfer grilles that are closed when facility is in use; * operated only when safety cabinets are not in use; MSC = microbiological safety cabinet

accidents or illness. Mirrors may be used to reflect areas that cannot be seen from outside the room.

Each TB level 3 room should have five clearly defined working areas:

(1) A reception bench for specimens.

(2) The cabinet bench with room either side for specimens before and cultures after processing in the cabinet.

(3) A staining area with a sink.

(4) A microscopy bench, preferably in the darker part of the room, especially if fluorescence microscopy is used.

(5) A 'clean' area for record keeping. As it is not good practice to keep papers and record books in level 3 laboratories, this area could be equipped with a computer terminal or a microphone system so that results and records may be transmitted to an office.

Floor spaces should be reserved for a centrifuge, incubator, refrigerator and an equipment cupboard. There should be a basin for hand washing (staff should not be expected to wash their hands in the sink used for staining slides), a cupboard for clean gowns and a linen bag for used gowns. Ideally these should all be in a lobby but, if this is not provided, they should be as near as possible to the door.

Microbiological safety cabinets

Although microbiological safety cabinets may be fitted in TB level 2 laboratories, they are essential at TB level 3. These cabinets differ fundamentally from chemical fume cupboards, which must not be accepted as a substitute for them. Arrangements for fitting microbiological safety cabinets should be made at the design stage. Afterthoughts usually result in poor performance and unnecessary expenditure.

There are three classes of microbiological safety cabinets but only Class I and Class II cabinets are suitable for the tuberculosis laboratory. They are both shown diagrammatically in Figure 2.4. In the Class I cabinet air at a velocity between 0.7 and 1.0 m/s passes in through the open front, and over the working area where it entrains any airborne bacteria and conveys them into the high efficiency particulate air (HEPA) filter which retains most, if not all, of them. It is then ducted to the outside of the building.

In the Class II cabinets air is also taken from the room and filtered but some is then recirculated vertically through the cabinet so that a 'curtain' of air descends across the working face and forms a barrier that prevents bacteria leaving or entering the cabinet. The remaining air is exhausted to outside the building.

In the United Kingdom there is an official preference for Class I cabinets for work with organisms in Risk Group III, but in the USA and much of the rest of the world Class II cabinets are the norm (Collins, 1993).

If a Class II microbiological safety cabinet is preferred then the 'thimble system' should be placed between the cabinet and the extractor fan (Figure 2.5). The thimble allows air to be extracted continuously from the room and from the safety cabinet when it is in use. Because of the differences in the velocities of air extracted from Class I and Class II cabinets thimble systems are not recommended for the former.

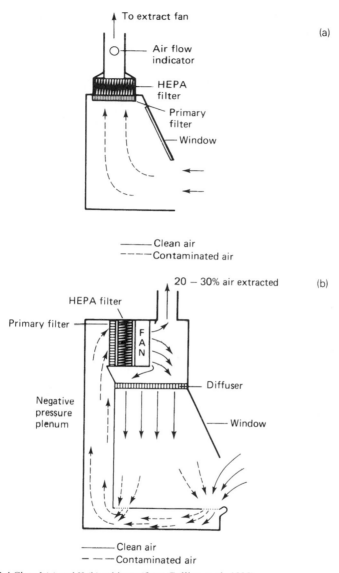

Figure 2.4 Class I (a) and II (b) cabinets (from Collins *et al.*, 1995)

Firm arrangements should be made for these cabinets to be installed correctly with due consideration given to airflow patterns and movements of people in the room. Performance tests and filter changes should be made regularly according to the national standard or the manufacturer's recommendations. For detailed information about the design, choice, siting, installation and testing of safety cabinets see Collins (1993). Safe techniques for using microbiological safety cabinets are given in Chapter 3, and procedures for decontaminating them in Chapter 4.

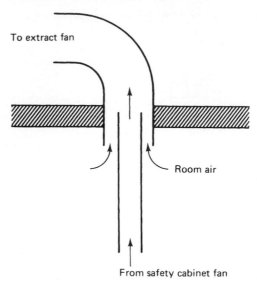

Figure 2.5 'Thimble' unit for a Class II microbiological safety cabinet. Arrows indicate direction of airflow (from Collins, 1993)

Laboratory equipment

Space does not permit a detailed inventory of equipment for every level of laboratory and this section is confined to listing the essential equipment for a TB level 3 laboratory. Advice on general equipment for work in level 2 laboratories is given by Cheesbrough (1984) and Collins *et al.* (1995). The large or expensive items are microbiological safety cabinets (see above), microscopes, autoclaves centrifuges, incubators and refrigerators.

Microscopes

Expensive and elaborate microscopes are unnecessary for tuberculosis bacteriology, but they should be binocular and comfortable to use as the worker may spend several hours with them every day. Microscopes, especially the fluorescence types, need regular maintenance. This should not be a problem in the larger laboratories but instruments provided for field work, many miles from the nearest instrument repairer, should be simple, robust and easily maintained by the staff of a peripheral laboratory. Such a laboratory may be equipped with only one microscope and therefore a spare oil immersion lens and spare eyepieces should be provided. Arrangements should be made for the prompt replacement of damaged optical equipment.

Autoclaves

An autoclave is necessary in all but the most remote laboratories. It need not be in the tuberculosis laboratory but should be nearby and in the same building. Ideally, separate autoclaves, one for sterilizing equipment and culture media and another for infectious waste, should be provided. Information about the use of autoclaves is given in Chapter 4.

Centrifuges

Centrifuges are essential in laboratories where tubercle bacilli are cultured (although as indicated on page 61 there are methods that do not involve centrifugation). The machine should be large enough to accept at least four buckets, each capable of holding one or more 28 ml screw-capped bottles ('universal containers'). Sealed buckets ('safety cups') should be provided. Sealed rotors are not recommended.

Incubators

Incubators are usually electrically operated, but oil-heated models are still available and have proved to be very reliable in places where there is no electricity supply. In large establishments walk-in incubators ('hot rooms') are more convenient. Problems arise in warm countries when incubation below the ambient temperature, e.g. for the identification of some mycobacteria, is required. Small incubators may be placed inside refrigerators, with the electricity supply taken in through a hole drilled through one of the walls. Alternatively, refrigerated incubators are available.

Refrigerators

Domestic-type refrigerators are adequate for most kinds of tuberculosis bacteriology but they should have a freezing compartment. Deep-freezers might be considered a luxury.

Bench equipment

Smaller equipment should include the following: slide staining racks; electrically heated drying racks; an electric slide heater; slide holders; a Vortex testtube mixer; a Waring type aerosol-free blender; Griffith or Ten Broeck glass-PTFE tissue grinders; alcohol-sand jars (autoclavable 500 ml jars containing 200 g sand and 250 ml alcohol for removing material from wire loops); hooded microbunsens; pipetting devices; an atomizer for disinfectant; diamond writing styli. Some pieces of small equipment are shown in Figure 2.6.

Research equipment

Equipment for chromatography and nucleic acid technology, etc. may be necessary in higher grade TB level 3 laboratories which have research programmes, but should be avoided in lower grade laboratories until it has been firmly established that they are cost-effective diagnostic tools.

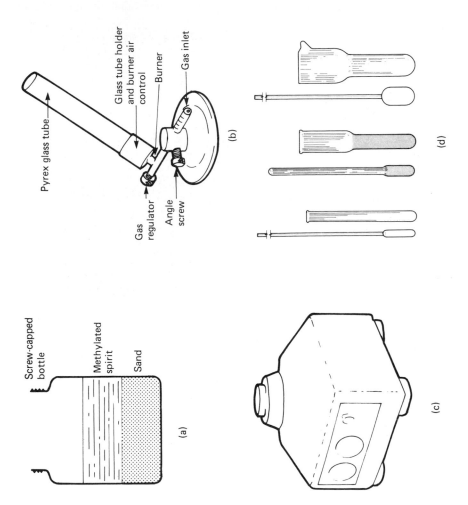

Pyrex glass tube

Glass tube holder and burner air control

Burner

Gas inlet

Gas regulator

Angle screw

(b)

(d)

Screw-capped bottle

Methylated spirit

Sand

(a)

(c)

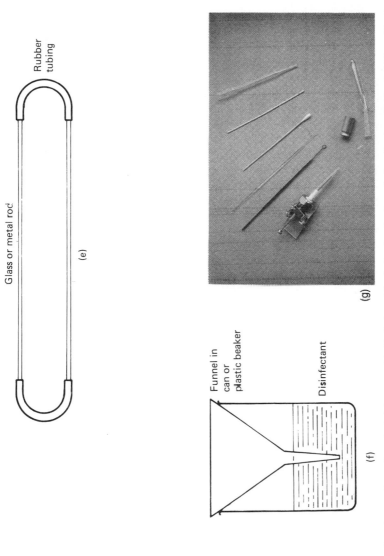

Glass or metal rod

Rubber tubing

(e)

Funnel in can or plastic beaker

Disinfectant

(f)

(g)

Figure 2.6 Small equipment for a tuberculosis laboratory. (a) Alcohol-sand bottle for cleaning loops before flaming. (b) Hooded (Kampff) microbunsen for safely flaming loops. (c) Vortex mixer. (d) Tissue homogenizers (Camlab). (e) Slide rack for staining. (f) Discard pot for pouring infected fluids into disinfectant. (g) Loops and pipetting aids

Training and motivation of staff

Training

Graduate microbiologists are rarely recruited directly into tuberculosis laboratories. They usually work for some time in clinical or research laboratories before they consider transferring. Serious 'in-service' training of newcomers, irrespective of their qualifications and experience in other fields, should begin at once, by apprenticing them to experienced workers. They should be taught, and gain considerable experience with, the basic techniques such as making and examining direct smears and preparing material for culture before they are allowed to embark on research or sophisticated investigations. Initial training should include instruction on laboratory-acquired tuberculosis and its prevention (Chapter 3).

Prospects for promotion in tuberculosis laboratories are not good and if young microbiologists have any ambitions it is usually necessary for them to move to other work in order to obtain wider experience and higher qualifications. The wastage is therefore high and only a small number of workers remain permanently dedicated to tuberculosis bacteriology.

Technical staff (technicians or technologists in some countries; medical laboratory scientific officers in the United Kingdom) may be employed at all levels from small peripheral laboratories to national reference centres. They usually obtain their qualifications by part-time or short-term attendance at colleges but some undertake longer courses leading to, for example, a Master of Science degree. The college courses are, however, tending to become more and more academic, to the detriment of good technical training which may then be obtained only if the laboratory in which they subsequently work maintains high standards. Unfortunately many senior technical staff are more concerned with 'management' than with good laboratory practice.

Tuberculosis bacteriology is just one of many activities with which technicians are involved and proper training in that field is usually deferred until they have two or three years of general experience and have obtained their initial qualifications. In the United Kingdom, for example, it is unusual for junior medical laboratory scientific officers to be employed in tuberculosis bacteriology. After they have obtained their first qualification they usually 'rotate' through the various laboratory departments or sections to gain experience for higher qualifications. This means that they may spend only a month or two in the tuberculosis laboratory and they may indeed never learn more than how to make direct smears and prepare cultures. Even when fully qualified, a technician may have to continue with the 'rotation' system rather than taking a full-time appointment in any one section.

The urge for promotion results in a fairly rapid turnover of staff and the permanent workers in tuberculosis laboratories spend a great deal of their time training people who move on as soon as they become reasonably competent. The American Thoracic Society (1983) recommended that technical staff should not rotate through tuberculosis laboratories but should remain committed to that particular type of work. For this recommendation to succeed, it is essential that such workers have similar job satisfaction (see below), salary scales and promotional prospects as their colleagues in other branches of clinical microbiology.

Laboratory assistants working in peripheral laboratories often have some experience in primary health care and at best will have received some training in an intermediate level laboratory. Often, though, training takes place at the peripheral laboratory itself, where it may vary from good to very bad. It should include the collection of good specimens, making smears of suitable material, staining and examining smears competently and the prompt dispatch of material to the nearest intermediate or central laboratory. Assistants should also be trained to service and repair equipment as the nearest service agent or instrument repairer may be hundreds of miles away. They should also be taught the simple management skills that ensure adequate stocks of materials are maintained (Mitchison, 1982).

Motivation

'Job satisfaction' is a well-known principle in management: people will perform well only if they are interested in their work it and find it psychologically, if not financially, rewarding. This is summed up in the word 'motivation'. There are no glib answers to the problems of staff motivation—or lack of it—in tuberculosis bacteriology. Our experience has taught us that only a few people really enjoy the work and for that reason alone it is often done badly outside those laboratories where there is enthusiasm and dedication and, above all, good leadership.

One outstanding reason why many people dislike working in a tuberculosis laboratory is that they have to manipulate sputum. Many years ago one of us was in charge of a laboratory where members of the staff often arrived late in the morning. He decreed that the last to arrive each day would do the sputum tests. This worked wonders for punctuality but did little for the quality of the tuberculosis work. Oddly enough, nobody ever objected to working with faeces, possibly because this material is 'natural' whereas sputum certainly is not.

Another cause of poor job satisfaction stems from the training programmes outlined above. Scientists and technicians who have spent four or five years obtaining their qualifications frequently resent doing what they consider to be menial tasks such as preparing and examining sputum smears. They look for what they imagine to be the glamour of research, particularly in 'molecular biology', or they prefer the excitement of the clinical laboratory where they may encounter and identify a dozen different organisms each day, often by 'kit' or automated methods that require little initiative or professional skill. Even if graduate and technical staff do adapt to what may appear to be mundane tasks and then progress and become more proficient at the more interesting work, such as identification and drug susceptibility testing of mycobacteria, they may not become sufficiently motivated to continue with it.

Motivation may be fostered in several ways. One is by associating all members of the laboratory staff with the clinical and epidemiological aspects of tuberculosis therapy and control. This may be achieved by arranging visits to clinics and hospitals, and talks and demonstrations by physicians. The laboratory staff should also be involved in clinical trials and contact tracing. All this will help them to appreciate the problems of tuberculosis at the 'sharp end' and make them feel valued members of a team. Another way of maintaining motivation and morale is to introduce a system of appraisal in which all members of staff meet with a senior person to discuss their career progress and any problems that they are likely to encounter. Properly conducted, this system identifies talents and abilities and also weaknesses so the former may be harnessed to mutual benefit and the latter addressed by suitable training. Unfortunately, this system, all too often, is run incompetently and in many centres the carrot of enthusiasm has been replaced by the stick of 'performance indicators'.

Whenever possible, all members of staff should be involved in some kind of research, whether as part of a team involved in a major project or on a small but useful technical exercise such as comparison of methods. Any contribution to research should be recognized when results are published, preferably by including the contributors as authors or at least by mentioning them in the acknowledgements.

Another problem relates to promotion. It is unfortunate that the highest paid jobs in the technical and scientific grades go not to those who have proved their worth at the laboratory bench but to those who hanker for the manager's chair and the committee room. This problem is unlikely to be resolved until there is a radical restructuring of career grades so that the best scientist or technician—and the distinction, as already suggested, is rapidly becoming blurred—can command the highest salary and status without having to engage in what is essentially the work of clerical and personnel assistants and store keepers.

In developing countries the problems of staff motivation, particularly in the peripheral laboratories, can be even more acute. The best qualified and motivated staff are likely to be concentrated in the central laboratories, with fewer at the intermediate level and perhaps none in the peripherals, which are the front line in the war against tuberculosis. The policy of sending technical staff from developing countries to the big city laboratories of the developed world results in their determination, whether or not they have acquired the skill, to do only the more sophisticated work and therefore to stay in their own big cities when they return home. Like some graduates and technicians in developed countries, they will claim that they have been trained for better things than sputum smears and cultures. The inevitable result is that the central laboratories become 'ivory towers' while the work at the peripheral, or even the intermediate, laboratories is left to the least skilled staff who are often poorly motivated. This results in a rapid turnover of staff at these levels and a poor quality of work.

Motivation of staff in peripheral laboratories needs different approaches as those suggested for the higher levels are mostly inappropriate. Health workers in the field cannot usually be expected to do any kind of research and may feel very much 'out on a limb'. Mitchison (1982) has suggested increased status and pay linked to an examination system. Those who pass would be awarded a certificate or diploma, the possession of which would enhance the personal standing and prestige of the health workers in their communities and motivate them to continue with the work.

Proficiency testing

Proficiency testing or quality control is highly desirable but not easy to achieve. Ideally, a central laboratory sends out natural or simulated specimens, some of which contain no acid-fast bacilli and others contain variable numbers. The recipients perform the investigations suitable to their level and report the results to the central laboratory which can then assess proficiency. In peripheral laboratories the ability of staff to prepare and examine sputum smears is assessed while at higher levels specimens will be cultured, species identified and drug susceptibility tests performed. With the introduction of new diagnostic methods such as nucleic acid probes and the polymerase chain reaction (PCR, p. 111) additional quality control systems will be required.

Participation in proficiency testing schemes may be compulsory or voluntary. In some countries, accreditation of laboratories requires participation in such schemes. Participation in voluntary schemes is more likely if the results remain confidential.

In the United Kingdom, which has a voluntary scheme, the quality assurance laboratory (QAL) of the Public Health Laboratory Service provides a variety of materials to participating laboratories who each have an identity code known only to themselves and the QAL. The QAL issues collective reports so that each of the participants can see how their proficiency compares with that of the others.

The College of American Pathologists has been conducting proficiency testing, geared to the Extent system, for many years, as well as surveys into methods used (Kubica *et al.*, 1975; Sommers and MacClatchy, 1983; Woods and Witebsky, 1995).

3

The prevention of laboratory-acquired tuberculosis

Laboratory-acquired tuberculosis has a long history and it is important that the risks of acquiring this disease and the precautions necessary to prevent, or at least minimize, such risks should take a prominent place in any laboratory manual that describes the methods for isolating and identifying tubercle bacilli and other mycobacteria.

Reports of both pulmonary and non-pulmonary laboratory-acquired tuberculosis have been reviewed and discussed by Collins (1993) and indicate the extent of the problem, despite attempts by various governments and organizations to prevent or at least minimize the risk (see, for example, Department of Health and Social Security 1970, 1978; Richmond and McKinney, 1993; Collins, 1993).

A number of non-pulmonary infections, resulting from cuts sustained during autopsies have also been reported (Grange *et al.*, 1988; Collins, 1993), as have laboratory-acquired infections with Bacille Calmette-Guérin (BCG) (Hollerström and Hard, 1953; Engbaek *et al.*, 1977).

The classification of mycobacteria on the basis of hazard

Various schemes exist for classifying micro-organisms into groups, classes or categories on the basis of the hazard they offer to those who work with them and to the community. That in current use in the European Union (Commission of the European Communities, 1990; Advisory Committee on Dangerous Pathogens, 1995) is shown in Table 3.1. Other states have adopted similar systems, e.g. that of World Health Organization (1993a). National guidelines may differ and should therefore be consulted.

In most systems members of the *Mycobacterium tuberculosis* complex are included in Hazard Group 3. There are differences, however, between the European Union and several other states and organizations concerning the position of certain other mycobacterial species, notably opportunist pathogens, which are variously listed in Groups 3 or 2 (Table 3.2). Mycobacteria not listed in either of these groups are presumed to be in Group 1. (There are no mycobacteria in Hazard Group 4.)

Containment or biosafety levels

Apart from design requirements, outlined in Chapter 2, the microbiological procedures used in the tuberculosis laboratory involve measures to minimize

Table 3.1 Classification of micro-organisms on the basis of hazard*

Group 1	A biological agent that is unlikely to cause human disease.
Group 2	A biological agent that can cause human disease and might be a hazard to workers; it is unlikely to spread to the community; there is usually effective prophylaxis and treatment available.
Group 3	A biological agent that can cause severe human disease and present a serious hazard to workers; it may present a risk of spreading to the community, but there is usually effective prophylaxis and treatment available.
Group 4†	A biological agent that causes severe human disease and is a serious hazard to workers; it may present a high risk of spreading to the community; there is usually no effective prophylaxis and treatment available.

*Commission of the European Communities (1990)
†There are no mycobacteria in Group 4

Table 3.2 Hazard groups of mycobacteria (species that are not listed are in hazard group 1)

Group 2	Group 3
M. asiaticum	M. tuberculosis
M. avium	M. bovis
M. chelonae	M. africanum
M. fortuitum	M. microti
M. haemophilum	M. leprae
M. intracellulare	
M. kansasii	
M. malmoense	
M. marinum	
M. paratuberculosis	
M. scrofulaceum	
M. shimoidei	
M. simiae	
M. szulgai	
M. ulcerans	
M. xenopi	

Based on the classification of the Commission of the European Union (1993).

airborne infection hazards as well as those intended to prevent infection by accidental ingestion and inoculation.

Airborne infection hazards

It is generally accepted that most of the workers who acquire tuberculosis in the laboratory become infected by inhaling airborne tubercle bacilli released during laboratory manipulations. A considerable measure of protection against such airborne infection is given by the controlled airflows in the level 3 containment laboratory and by microbiological safety cabinets but neither of these is a substitute for good technique. Nor will they protect the worker against a massive release of airborne bacilli or contact with spilled infectious material.

Many microbiological techniques generate aerosols (Collins, 1993). These are minute droplets of liquid that are formed when bubbles burst and other thin films of liquid are separated. They are also formed when liquids are squirted through small orifices, impinge on surfaces (even of other liquids) and during pipetting and pouring operations They are generated in large amounts when tubes containing liquids break during centrifugation. Each droplet may contain one or more micro-organism. The smaller droplets (those less than 5 μm in diameter) settle very slowly and dry rapidly, leaving the organisms they contain as 'droplet nuclei' or infective airborne particles. These particles float in the air of a room and are moved about by even quite small air currents. If inhaled, they may reach the alveoli and initiate an infection. Larger droplets settle rapidly and may contaminate surfaces, the hands and clothing.

Measures that reduce, or at least minimize, the generation of aerosols and airborne infectious particles are considered below.

Work with bacteriological loops

Vigorous spreading of infected material during the preparation of smears for microscopy and in the inoculation of culture media should be avoided. Loops should be used gently. Saturated mercuric chloride, not saline or water, should be used for making films of cultures as this kills tubercle bacilli rapidly. Loops charged with infectious material should not be placed in the flames of ordinary Bunsen burners as the material may spatter before it is burned and thus contaminate surfaces. Loops should first be cleaned by rotating them in an alcohol-sand bath or they should be held in the flame of a hooded microbunsen (Figure 2.6, p. 20). Disposable plastic loops are better than wire loops.

Pipetting

Pipettes should be drained, not blown out violently, or the last drop will form bubbles which burst and form aerosols. Pasteur pipettes are particularly likely to generate bubbles. Pipetting devices (essential, as mouth pipetting must not be permitted) should be selected with care as some of them expel the pipette contents with some force.

Opening culture bottles and plates

If there is a thin film of fluid between the rim of the bottle and its cap, or between the rim and lid of a Petri dish, aerosols will be formed when they are separated. Bottles and dishes containing mycobacterial cultures should always be opened in a safety cabinet.

Centrifugation

Fluid will spill from uncapped centrifuge tubes and be aerosolized by the action of the rotor in the bowl. Such aerosols will be ejected with considerable velocity through the gap between the lid and the bowl and through the ventilation ports. Even if tubes are capped there is a risk that one will break, releasing a large amount of aerosol. Sealed centrifuge buckets (Figure 3.1) should always be used in tuberculosis laboratories and the usual precautions taken to ensure that opposing buckets are correctly balanced and that they sit securely in their trunnions.

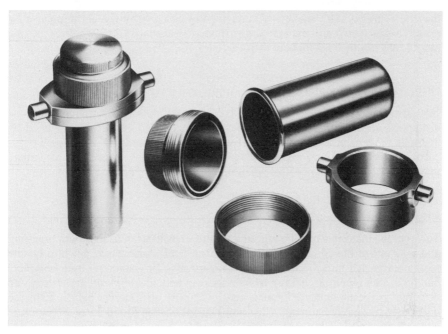

Figure 3.1 Sealed centrifuge buckets ('safety cups'). Available with polycarbonate or metal screw-in caps (MSE) (from Collins, 1993)

Mechanical homogenizers

These are used to homogenize sputum and other materials, thereby facilitating decontamination. Some instruments leak at the seals and release aerosols. Homogenizers should be covered during use with plastic boxes, which are disinfected afterwards. They should not be opened immediately after use, as aerosols are generated during the process. A few minutes should elapse before they are opened in a microbiological safety cabinet.

Pouring into disinfectant

When infectious material is poured into disinfectant it may splash and contaminate the surrounding surfaces and may produce aerosols. The apparatus shown in Figure 2.6 should be used. The end of the funnel should be beneath the surface of the disinfectant in the jar or can and the material to be discarded poured carefully down the side of the funnel. Pouring the contents of a container will inevitably contaminate the rim. This should be wiped with a piece of disinfectant-soaked filter paper which is then discarded into the bench discard jar.

Reciprocating shakers

These are used in some laboratories to assist in homogenization and decontamination of sputum. Unless the bottle or tube caps are screwed on securely aerosols may be released. The shakers should, in any case, be covered during use by plastic boxes which are afterwards disinfected. Alternatively, the bottles may be placed into plastic bags that are then sealed.

Dispersal of dried material

Not all infectious airborne particles arise from aerosols. Dried material may be dispersed, for example, when ampoules of freeze-dried cultures are opened by methods other than those prescribed by the issuing laboratory. Dried pathological material and sputum homogenates around the screw threads of containers may be released as fine powders when the containers are opened.

Ingestion hazards

Tuberculous materials may be ingested by direct aspiration as in mouth pipetting and by putting fingers and articles that have been contaminated while on the laboratory bench into the mouth. This hazard may be overcome by a complete ban on mouth pipetting, licking labels, sucking pencils, smoking and eating and drinking in the laboratory. Fingers may also pick up tubercle bacilli from the outside of sputum containers. Allen and Darrell (1983) found 18 of 279 sputum containers (6.5%) were contaminated in this way. It may be necessary to disinfect containers as a routine measure.

Inoculation hazards

'Needlestick' accidents, in which staff are accidentally stabbed by hypodermic needles which may be infected, are regrettably common. Syringes and needles should not be used as substitutes for pipettes as there are many safer devices on the market for the measurement of small amounts of fluid. Cuts from infected glassware also occur and, in this respect, glass Pasteur pipettes are the most dangerous objects. The soft plastic varieties are much safer. Scalpels and other sharps used to prepare tissues also offer a hazard. Needlestick accidents and other injuries acquired in the laboratory should be reported to the relevant occupational health department.

Glass tissue homogenizers (Figure 2.6) may break during use, resulting in cut hands and fingers. Gloves should therefore be worn and the instruments be held in a wad of disinfectant-soaked cottonwool.

Work in microbiological safety cabinets

Microbiological safety cabinets are intended to protect the worker from inhalation of aerosols or other infected airborne particles that may be inadvertently released during manipulations or as a result of accidents. Some also protect the work from contaminants in room air.

The two classes of cabinet, I and II, normally used in tuberculosis laboratories, are described in Chapter 2.

The following precautions and technical procedures are recommended for manipulations with infected material in microbiological safety cabinets.

- After switching on the exhaust fan, the worker should not commence work until a safe airflow is established, as indicated by the meter or the audible warning signal.
- All necessary equipment should be placed in the cabinet before work is commenced. If it is necessary to remove and replace equipment and materials, work should not be recommenced until adequate airflow is re-established, as indicated by the meter. Removing the hands and arms from the cabinet will disturb, and may compromise, the safety of the airflow.
- All work should be conducted well within the cabinet. It is advisable to place a strip of tape (e.g. yellow Biohazard tape), across the front of the working area and approximately 150 mm from the front edge (behind the grille on a Class II cabinet) beyond which all work should be conducted.
- Traditional Bunsen burners should not be used as the hot air from them will compromise the air flow and may damage the filters. Hooded microbunsens (Figure 2.6) may be used if it is first ascertained that they have no adverse effect on the air flow, but it is best to use plastic inoculation loops which are discarded into disinfectant after use.
- Tall pipette jars should not be used unless they can be placed at an angle (Figure 3.2). They should be made of plastic, not glass. Alternatively, pipettes may be discarded into instrument (e.g. catheter) trays containing disinfectant.
- When work is finished, arms and articles should not be removed immediately from the cabinet. The cabinet should be left running for several minutes to permit removal of aerosols.

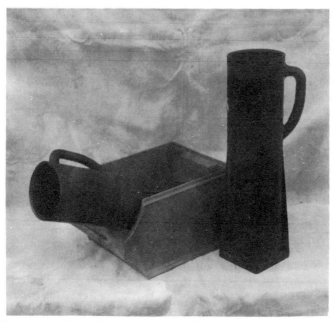

Figure 3.2 Pipette jars. Rubber and polypropylene are safer than glass. Sloping jars are safer and more convenient than those that are used upright (from Collins, 1993)

Personal precautions

Laboratory workers should maintain high standards of personal hygiene and, in particular, wash their hands frequently and certainly after removing any protective clothing and before leaving the room. Any cuts or abrasions on exposed skin surfaces should be covered with waterproof dressings.

Personal outdoor clothing, shopping bags and other articles that will be taken home should be placed in lockers outside the containment laboratory.

Protective clothing should be worn at all times. The choice is between gowns of the operating-room type or coats that wrap over the body, fasten at the side and cover the upper chest and neck. Sleeves should be wrist length and gathered to prevent contamination of the sleeves of normal clothing and to prevent particles entering the sleeves when the worker is using a safety cabinet. Protective clothing should be removed before the wearer leaves the containment laboratory.

Disposable gloves, of the good quality surgical variety, should be available in various sizes and workers should be encouraged to wear them when they handle infected material. Surgeons' masks are not necessary as they offer little protection and give a false sense of security.

Medical supervision

Staff who work with tubercle bacilli should be healthy and well nourished. They should have a pre-employment medical examination and chest radiograph. Policies for BCG vaccination vary from country to country. In the United Kingdom, BCG is offered to those who are negative on tuberculin testing unless there is definite evidence of previous vaccination. Those requiring BCG vaccination should be excluded from the tuberculosis laboratory until they have been vaccinated.

Regular, e.g. annual, medical examinations by occupational health physicians are advisable. The use of annual chest radiography is controversial on account of the radiation hazard. Reliance is now usually placed on instructing staff to seek medical advice if they develop symptoms such as a chronic cough. Symptom surveys, based on suitable questionnaires, may also be used. For information on the role of occupational health services in the prevention and control of tuberculosis among hospital workers, including laboratory staff, see George (1988).

4

Sterilization, disinfection and the disposal of infected waste

The words sterilization and disinfection do not have the same meaning. Sterilization implies the complete destruction of all organisms; disinfection implies the inactivation of micro-organisms, including those capable of causing disease but not necessarily bacterial spores (and certain viruses), on the surfaces of inanimate objects (Russell, 1996). In laboratories, sterilization is usually accomplished by autoclaving and disinfection by treatment with chemicals.

Autoclaving

Autoclaving is the optimal initial procedure for sterilizing equipment and culture media and for making infected material safe for disposal. Staff should be carefully instructed in the procedures. Autoclaves should be tested periodically to ensure that the temperature achieved in the chamber is high enough to kill all bacteria. The minimum temperature should be 121 °C and this should be maintained for 15 minutes. Testing is best done by placing thermocouples in the load and connecting them to an external recorder. If these instruments are not available, sterilizer indicator tubes are the best alternative. These are placed in the load and are examined when the autoclave is opened after use. The indicator changes colour if the process is adequate (the range of colours is given by the manufacturers).

The autoclaves for levels 2 and 3 laboratories are usually of the conventional type, as shown in Figure 4.1. and may or may not have steam jackets. The material to be sterilized is placed in the chamber and the door is tightly closed. Air is removed, either by downward displacement by steam or by an exhaust pump, and steam at high pressure is admitted.

The higher the pressure, the higher the temperature. The material is exposed for a predetermined time; the final temperature/time combination required to achieve sterilization is usually 121 °C for 15–20 minutes, but some modern automated autoclaves operate at 134 °C for 3–5 minutes.

When the cycle is complete, the steam is exhausted from the chamber and the contents are cooled, either by water or air, and when the temperature has fallen to below 80 °C the door of the autoclave may be opened and the contents removed.

The temperature in the chamber is measured by thermocouples and recorded on a chart. In some old autoclaves the temperature probe is placed in the drain and gives much higher (and therefore misleading) readings than those in the

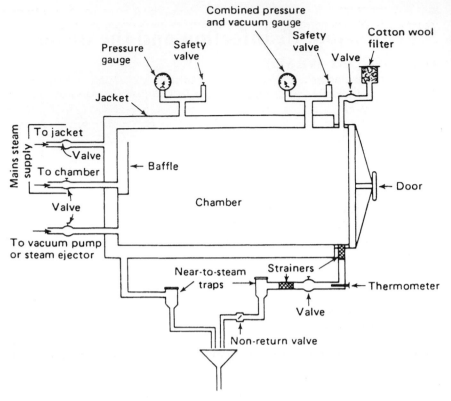

Figure 4.1 Gravity displacement autoclave (from Collins *et al.*, 1995)

chamber, leading to a reduction in holding time and therefore a failure to sterilize. In most modern autoclaves the sterilizing cycles are automatically controlled to preset conditions.

For further information about laboratory autoclaves and autoclaving see Russell *et al.* (1992) and Collins (1993).

Disinfectants and disinfection

Chemical disinfectants used in tuberculosis bacteriology include phenolics, hypochlorites, alcohols and aldehydes.

Phenolics
It is generally accepted that the disinfectants most active against tubercle bacilli and other mycobacteria are the phenolics, among which there are various formulations, e.g. Sudol, Printol, Clearsol. Phenolic disinfectants should be diluted accurately according to the manufacturers' instructions for 'dirty or worst possible situations'. The dilutions should be freshly prepared each day as their activity diminishes on storage.

Phenolics, suitably diluted, are used in bench discard jars, pipette jars and other containers for small items of equipment and waste. The articles must come into intimate contact with the fluid. No air bubbles should be seen in submerged objects. The contact period should be at least 18 hours (usually overnight).

Hypochlorites
Although hypochlorites are also effective against the mycobacteria themselves, they are more readily inactivated by materials containing protein, e.g. by sputum. They are therefore not normally used in tuberculosis bacteriology laboratories, although they are the disinfectants of choice for specimens from HIV-positive patients.

Alcohol
Alcohol, usually 70% ethanol (methylated spirit), or propanol, is used in alcohol-sand baths and for decontaminating benches, safety cabinet work surfaces and centrifuge bowls. For these purposes it is convenient to use a domestic or horticultural sprayer. Alcohol should also be used instead of water to balance centrifuge buckets.

Aldehydes
Glutaraldehyde kills mycobacteria but is now recognized as offering a health hazard. Formaldehyde (gas) and formalin (an aqueous solution of the gas) are also effective but, as they are toxic, their use is best restricted to space disinfection ('fumigation'), e.g. of microbiological safety cabinets and rooms (see below).

Personal precautions with disinfectants
All these disinfectants are toxic and exposure may result in respiratory distress, skin rashes or conjunctivitis. Eye and face protection, and gloves, should be worn during the dilution of bulk disinfectants.

For further information on laboratory disinfectants see Russell (1996), Russell *et al.* (1992) and Collins (1993).

Disposal of infected materials and waste

It is essential that all infected waste arising from work in clinical laboratories is made safe to handle by autoclaving before disposal by incineration.

All pathological material, smears, cultures and the vessels in which they were grown should be sterilized or (exceptionally) disinfected before re-use or disposal. It is unsafe to send infected laboratory waste for off-site incineration, e.g. by transport on the public highway (Collins, 1994).

Containers for infected waste

Primary containers for the collection and disposal of infected waste include metal or thermoresistant plastic bins or buckets, plastic bags, 'sharps' containers, and bench discard jars.

Bins and buckets
These may be circular, square or rectangular in section but not more than 25 cm deep or there may be problems with steam penetration. They should fit the autoclave chamber loosely, so that there is at least a 10 cm space all round them, again to permit the free passage of steam.

Plastic bags
These are usually colour coded. In the United Kingdom those intended for waste which will be autoclaved are light blue in colour, as BS standard colour No. 175 (British Standards Institution, 1988), or transparent with a light blue inscription 'Waste for Autoclaving' and bearing the international biohazard sign (Figure 4.2). Bags intended for the incineration of waste after it has been autoclaved are opaque and yellow in colour, as BS standard colour No. 309 (British Standards Institution, 1988), with the printed words 'Waste for Incineration Only' and the international biohazard sign.

There appears to be no official specification for the strength or thickness (gauge) of plastic for these bags but a thickness of 25 μm for high density polyethylene for waste of low to intermediate risk and 100 μm for high density polyethylene for high level risk material has been suggested (Sims, 1991).

Blue or transparent bags, containing material for autoclaving, should be supported during use in rigid or plastic containers to avoid bursting. The bags must not be filled to capacity; about one third capacity is ideal as they will be closed and securely fastened before removal for sterilization. For this purpose plastic ties are used but are removed before the bags are consigned to the autoclave to avoid problems with steam penetration. In some of the modern autoclaves that operate at a high temperature and pressure the bags may remain sealed. Tests should be performed for each laboratory autoclave to determine whether bags may be sealed. Use of sealed bags diminishes the chances of release of infectious material.

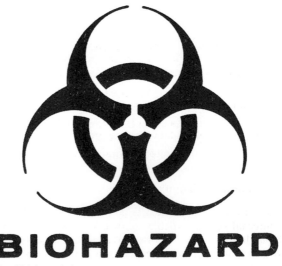

BIOHAZARD

Figure 4.2 International biohazard sign

It is likely that there will soon be a move away from plastic bags in favour of the more rigid disposable containers that are used for certain anatomical material (e.g. amputations), such as the single-use polyethylene drums as used in certain European states (German DIN Standard V 30 739). As such containers will be incinerated they must not be made of polyvinyl chloride (PVC) to avoid the risk of the formation of dioxins if the incinerator is operated at suboptimal temperatures.

'Sharps' containers
There is a British Standard (British Standards Institution, 1990) for containers for hollow-bore needles, slides and other sharp objects used in health care and laboratories. These containers, yellow in colour and made of rigid plastic capable of being incinerated, must be puncture-resistant and leak-proof, even if roughly handled, and provided with handles. The aperture should permit the easy, single-handed, insertion of the waste article without external contamination, but will not permit removal of the contents. Each container must be clearly marked 'Danger: Contaminated Sharps only; To be incinerated'. There should also be a horizontal mark indicating three-quarters of the total volume, marked 'Do not fill above this line'.

Bench discard jars
These jars or pots contain chemical disinfectants and are intended for the reception of small infected items of bench equipment such as Pasteur pipettes and similar waste generated during microbiological manipulations. They should be made of robust autoclavable plastic, about 1000 ml in capacity and only two-thirds filled with the disinfectant. The best kind of discard jar can be closed after use with a screw cap so that the jar may be inverted to remove air bubbles and bring all the contents into contact with the disinfectant.

Some laboratories use 'sharps' containers instead of bench discard jars, with or without disinfectant.

Treatment and disposal

After autoclaving, the blue or transparent bags containing the waste material should be placed in yellow bags and sent for incineration. In the United Kingdom, some waste regulatory authorities will permit autoclaved waste to be sent for landfill, in which case yellow bags with black stripes should be used.

When disinfectants are used, the contact period should be not less than 18 hours (usually overnight). The fluid should then be poured away and the disinfected articles autoclaved and/or incinerated. The containers should then be washed in very hot water.

Decontamination of microbiological safety cabinets

Microbiological safety cabinets must be decontaminated (disinfected) regularly. The exposed internal surfaces of the cabinet working space may be decontaminated with 70% alcohol. This is safer to use than glutaraldehyde and is just as effective if it is left in contact with the surface overnight. Cabinets should be decontaminated daily, or after each working session. The most effective method is spraying from a plastic hand-held sprayer or 'atomizer' of the kind used in homes and gardens.

The whole cabinet, including the inaccessible parts such as the plenum and the filters in their housings must be decontaminated before maintenance and filter changes. Formaldehyde is the usual disinfectant (see the warnings about aldehydes, above).

The usual procedure is to boil formalin and water to release formaldehyde. The water is necessary to maintain a relative humidity of about 70%, at which the gas has the maximum antimicrobial effect.

- A mixture of formalin and water, 25 ml of each, is placed in a small pan fitted with a thermal cut-out in the cabinet (in some cabinets this is built in).
- The front closure of the cabinet is fitted and sealed with tape if necessary. The pan heater is then switched on.
- When about half the volume of formalin has evaporated, the cabinet fan is switched on for 10–15 seconds to allow the gas to reach the filters.
- When all the formalin has evaporated the fan is switched on again for 10–15 seconds.
- Not less than 6 hours later the front closure is opened slightly and the extract fan switched on to purge the cabinet of formaldehyde.
- Five minutes later the front closure is removed and the cabinet fan run for 30 minutes to exhaust the remaining formaldehyde to the external atmosphere.

This method works well with safety cabinets that exhaust to atmosphere outside the building. Problems arise when cabinets are permitted to recirculate air to laboratory rooms. It may then be necessary to seal the room during the operation, which may take up to 24 hours. Modifications have been made to Class II cabinets, especially in Australia (Standards Association of Australia, 1983), that enable the gas to be recirculated through the cabinet during the decontamination cycle, but there still remains the problem of disposal or neutralization of the residual formaldehyde. The extracted air may also be passed through alumina to remove formaldehyde (for details of methods for neutralizing formalin, see p. 40).

It is now generally accepted that the generation of formaldehyde by mixing paraformaldehyde with potassium permanganate is an unsafe procedure as in certain proportions the mixture is explosive.

Decontamination of laboratory rooms

Level 3 laboratories must be sealable so that they may be disinfected without harm to other occupants of the building (Advisory Committee on Dangerous Pathogens, 1995). This assumes that the agent used will be formaldehyde which, as indicated above, is a hazardous substance. Fortunately it is rarely necessary to fumigate tuberculosis laboratories with formaldehyde. The occasions when it may be necessary are after accidents in which large amounts of cultures are spilled or dispersed, and before the laboratory is decommissioned for maintenance or other work necessitating the entry of non-laboratory staff.

Fumigation of rooms with formaldehyde should never be undertaken lightly and, if local staff are not experienced, it is wise to consult other, more experienced people about the suitability of the premises and the exact procedure to be used.

It is essential that a risk assessment is made before formaldehyde is used. The hazards offered by fumigation may be greater than those presented by simple cleaning up and using a phenolic compound.

A prerequisite for formaldehyde disinfection of rooms is respiratory protective equipment (RPE). Canister-type respirators are unsuitable for this purpose and positive-pressure self-contained breathing apparatus (SCBA) should be used. SCBA should be tested at regular intervals and users should receive intensive initial training and refresher training at specified intervals.

Formaldehyde decontamination
The following methods are summarized from various published sources (Cheney and Collins, 1995; Jones, 1995). The procedure is essentially designed for planned decontamination and may have to be modified locally in case of emergency. Formaldehyde will damage computerized equipment which should therefore be removed from the area to be decontaminated.

- For each 30 m^3 of space, 100 ml of formalin plus 900 ml of water are required along with a suitable electric boiler. Self-adhesive sealing tape is used to seal around door jambs, windows and pipe ducts. In rooms that are more difficult to seal, polythene sheeting may also be required. This equipment should be stored in a readily accessible place, but not in the room for which it may be required.
- Two people are required; each should be experienced in the both the technique and the use of SCBA.
- Notice should be given to all staff and management that the room is to be decontaminated. Any smoke or fire detectors should be inactivated and mechanical ventilation isolated.
- All chlorine-containing chemicals, e.g. hypochlorite disinfectants, should be removed to avoid the possible formation of *bis* (chloromethyl) ether — a known carcinogen.
- One person should enter the room to carry out any sealing that may be required and to place the formaldehyde and water in the boiler. The second person remains available outside in case problems arise. If the room is being fumigated because of a hazardous spill, any obvious material should be cleared up with a suitable liquid disinfectant as the formaldehyde vapour is unlikely to be effective against any protein-containing materials, such as culture media, which will protect micro-organisms from the action of the fumigant.
- The boiler is then switched on and the operator must leave the room. It is useful to have a boiler with a cut-out which will operate when all the liquid has boiled away, or a time switch may be used. In the design of new rooms that are intended to be easily fumigated it is useful to have an electrical socket outlet which can be operated from outside the room.
- The exit door is then sealed and a large notice 'Room sealed for fumigation, (date and time)' is displayed in a prominent place.
- If a sampling port is built into the room, the concentration of formaldehyde gas may be monitored at intervals during the fumigation period.
- Not less than 12 hours later, the fumigant is removed from the room by turning on the microbiological safety cabinet or ventilation system from outside the room. If this cannot be done from outside the room then one operator, wearing SCBA, must enter the room to turn on the cabinets.

It is desirable that the formaldehyde concentration in the air is measured by one of the commercially available instruments. The reading should not be more than 2.5 mg/m^3 but even this will still be detectable by the majority of people and if mechanical ventilation is shut off or windows are closed the level in the room will rise again. This occurs because formaldehyde is absorbed to many surfaces during the fumigation process and it also polymerizes on to other surfaces. This absorption and polymerization, along with small, often undetectable, leaks that occur despite the sealing materials and the tendency of the gas to dissolve in condensation on surfaces cause the actual levels of formaldehyde in the room during the fumigation period to be lower than those which would be predicted by calculation. The absorbed and polymerized material can subsequently release formaldehyde over a period of time, causing the concentration of the gas in the room to reach detectable levels. This can be distressing to people who have to work there. A tray containing a cloth soaked in a strong or saturated solution of sodium sulphite will absorb residual formaldehyde and lower the levels. Walls may be washed with sodium sulphite solution if necessary. In view of this, it is sensible to construct the laboratory with the minimum of material likely to absorb formaldehyde and to use paint that will minimize absorption into walls and also be easily washable.

For more detailed information about formaldehyde decontamination and the hazards involved see Cheney and Collins (1995) and Jones (1995). Information on appropriate respiratory protection equipment is given by Harrington *et al.* (1992).

5

Collection, preservation and transport of specimens

Tubercle bacilli or other mycobacteria may be present in almost any pathological material but success in finding them in microscopic preparations and cultures depends initially on the care taken in selecting and collecting the specimens.

Essential prerequisites for the safe collection of satisfactory specimens are the containers which should be sterile, robust and leakproof.

Collection of specimens

Sputum

In spite of the wide variety of glass, plastic and metal jars, pots and bottles that are available, no really satisfactory sputum container exists. If the patient is to produce sputum directly into the container it must have a wide mouth, otherwise the outside will certainly become contaminated. Wide-mouthed containers, however, are difficult to stopper. Screw-on caps easily become cross-threaded; large press-on lids become distorted and the wads or liners in both kinds frequently fall out. In any case, the contents will leak and may contaminate the hands or person of anyone who handles them. In hot climates and when the specimen has to travel some distance, the contents of improperly closed containers are likely to dry up before they can be examined.

When there is a choice, the least unsatisfactory containers are glass or plastic pots 5–6 cm deep with 4–5 cm diameter mouths. Plastic pots suitable for use in developing countries may be obtained from UNICEF. These are easily burned after use. It is good practice to supply patients with plastic bags in which they can place their specimen containers before sending or taking them to the laboratory.

Sputum is the specimen of choice in the investigation of pulmonary disease and should be collected whenever possible, preferably before commencement of chemotherapy.

It is best to collect the first specimen at the clinic. The health worker can explain why the specimen is needed and that sputum, coughed up from deep in the lungs is required, not saliva. The patient should be instructed to place the container against the lower lip and to expectorate carefully so that the outside of the container is not contaminated.

Not all patients can cough up sputum from the lower respiratory tract at their first attempt; supervision and encouragement by the nurse, physiotherapist, technician or laboratory assistant not only ensures that a good first specimen is obtained, but that subsequent specimens, preferably collected early in the morning on each of the next two days, are also satisfactory. Sputum may be induced by inhalation of nebulized twice normal (hypertonic) saline for 5–15 minutes. Sputum, whether induced or not, should be collected away from susceptible patients; mini-epidemics of tuberculosis among HIV-positive patients have been traced to the encouragement of heavy coughing in clinics and open wards for the purpose of producing sputum for examination. Where weather permits, sputum may be collected in the open air. A good specimen for laboratory examination should be between 2 and 5 ml.

At least three consecutive daily sputum specimens may be necessary for diagnosis as tubercle bacilli are released intermittently from lesions in the lungs. Three specimens give a 95% chance of recovery of tubercle bacilli. Specimens should not be pooled: this could dilute a positive sample, distribute contaminants and also introduce problems in preparing cultures.

Patients should be asked not to clean their teeth or to use antiseptic mouth washes just before providing a sputum specimen.

Laryngeal swabs and gastric aspiration

Expectorated sputum is by far the best material for the diagnosis of pulmonary tuberculosis but if this cannot be obtained the much less effectual procedures of laryngeal swabbing and gastric aspiration may be used. Laryngeal swabs provide material for culture but they are almost useless for direct smear microscopy. The swabs are made of stiff wire, about 25 cm long and bent at one end to give an angle of about 35 degrees. This end is roughened with a file so that the cotton wool swab, not more than 0.5 cm thick, may be wound on tightly and will not become detached in the patient's larynx. Bicycle spokes, which have a screw thread at one end, make excellent laryngeal swabs. The swabs are placed in glass tubes, with about 5 cm of the straight end protruding; the tubes are plugged with cotton wool and sterilized. Some laboratories issue swabs tipped with alginate wool which can subsequently be dissolved so as to liberate the mycobacteria. Two swabs should be taken from each patient by a physician or trained nurse who is skilled in visualizing the larynx, and who should wear a visor because the patient will cough violently when the swab is inserted into the throat.

Gastric aspiration is performed in the morning before food or drink is taken. The patient is instructed to cough and swallow several times, after which the stomach contents are aspirated through a nasogastric tube. As the aspirate contains hydrochloric acid from the stomach, which may kill mycobacteria, the specimen should be taken immediately to the laboratory or neutralized with sodium hydroxide.

Bronchoscopy and transtracheal aspiration

The fibreoptic bronchoscope is being used increasingly to obtain specimens from the respiratory tract. It is used to take biopsies of radiological opacities, to harvest material on the bronchial walls by means of a small extensible brush and to wash sections of the bronchial tree with saline (broncho-alveolar lavage).

After use, the bronchoscope is sterilized with a 2% solution of glutaraldehyde. Inadequate sterilization of bronchoscopes, or subsequent washing with water containing environmental mycobacteria, has led to 'false' positive bacteriological reports (Gubler *et al.*, 1992; Kiely *et al.*, 1995) and is a potential cause of transmission of disease.

Descriptions of the clinical procedures of bronchoscopy are outside the scope of this book. Our personal experience, however, is that the Lukan traps used in the collection of bronchoscopy specimens and bronchial lavage fluid are highly unsuitable specimen containers. They are particularly liable to leak and frequently arrive at the laboratory in a messy and unsatisfactory condition.

Transtracheal aspiration is a risky procedure which is distressing to the patients. It has now been almost entirely superseded by fibreoptic bronchoscopy.

Urine

The most satisfactory containers for urine specimens are the 28 ml straight-sided screw-capped glass or plastic bottles known as universal containers. One advantage of these is that they fit 50 ml centrifuge buckets, obviating transfer of fluid to centrifuge tubes. Twenty-four hour specimens should be discouraged; they usually become contaminated. Preservatives, added to 24-hour urine containers for biochemical investigations, may render tubercle bacilli uncultivable. Some laboratories isolate mycobacteria by membrane filtration of total early-morning specimens.

The best results are obtained from early morning midstream specimens. Women may have difficulties with these containers and should be instructed to pass a midstream specimen into a wide-mouthed vessel which has been boiled and to fill the specimen bottle from that vessel. Three consecutive daily specimens should be provided.

Aspirated fluids and pus

Again, the 28 ml screw-capped universal containers are ideal. Plain bottles and bottles containing a non-bactericidal anticoagulant should be provided for the collection of aspirated fluids. Plain bottles are suitable for pus and exudates. Examination of cerebrospinal fluid is an emergency procedure: the laboratory staff should be alerted by the clinician and the specimen delivered without delay.

Fluids that are likely to form clots should be divided between two bottles, one plain and the other containing citrate or some other non-bactericidal anticoagulant. Alternatively, these fluids may be added directly to an equal quantity of a double-strength liquid medium e.g. Kirchner or Middlebrook 7H9 broth.

Samples for cytological and chemical examination may also be required and should be placed in separate containers.

As much pus as possible should be collected into a plain bottle. Throat swabs dipped in pus are rarely satisfactory specimens for tuberculosis bacteriology and should be regarded as a last resort and used only when a very small amount of material can be obtained. Transport medium (Kirchner or Middlebrook 7H9 broth) should then be used.

Tissue

Tissue is preferable to necrotic material or pus, as the latter contain free fatty acids that are toxic to mycobacteria. Universal containers, sputum pots or larger glass jars may be used, depending on the size of the specimen. The containers used for histological specimens should not be used. The fixative kills tubercle bacilli and even if this is poured off enough may remain to affect bacteriological examination.

Collection is the province of the surgeons, but they should be persuaded to divide the material between the microbiologist and the histopathologist and not expect both to work with the same material.

Blood

Between 5 and 25 ml of venous blood should be collected in 28 ml screw-capped bottles containing a non-bactericidal anticoagulant. Alternatively blood may be collected directly into blood culture bottles (see Chapter 7, p. 63).

Milk samples (from cows)

Screw-capped bottles, at least 100 ml capacity, should be provided. About 100 ml should be collected from each teat. Foremilk may be included. Samples from bulk milk containers are useless.

Water

Water is occasionally examined for opportunist mycobacteria, e.g. in tracing contamination. At least 2 litres should be collected in sterile screw-capped winchester bottles.

Identifying specimens

The container should be labelled at the time the specimen is collected. If it is labelled earlier it may be used by someone else; if labelled later it may be confused with the specimen of another patient. The patient's name and some other identification such as the clinic or hospital number, and the date and time of collection, should be written clearly on the label. Hospitals and clinics frequently have several patients with the same names.

Request forms

The specimen should be accompanied by a request form completed, or at least signed, by the doctor requesting the examination. The laboratory should provide sensible forms and those who make requests should write legibly and give the information required. The request form should ask for the minimum of information. The more questions asked the less likely they are to be answered.

The information required by the laboratory is:

• The name of the person or organization requesting the test and who expects to receive the report.

- The address to which the report should be sent.
- The surname or family name of the patient, followed by his/her given or local name.
- Some other identification of the patient, e.g. hospital or clinic number.
- The sex and age or date of birth of the patient.
- The nature of the specimen, e.g. sputum, urine, pleural fluid. If the specimen is pus or tissue, the site from which it came must be stated.
- The date and time of collection of the specimen.
- The examination required.
- Diagnosis or very brief clinical information.

Failure to give the required information in this list is discourteous and may indicate a low standard of care, especially when specimens or cultures are sent from one laboratory to another. There may be some problems in developing countries in supplying names and ages but in developed countries, where medical records are or should be in good order, there is no excuse.

Preservation of specimens

In the laboratory specimens may be preserved for several weeks in a refrigerator, preferably at or just below 0 °C. Preservation during transport at ambient temperatures requires chemical treatment. Three methods give reasonably good results:

- The fresh specimen is mixed with an equal volume of 1% cetyl pyridinium chloride (or bromide) in 2% sodium chloride solution. Tubercle bacilli will survive in this for at least a week.
- The fresh specimen is mixed with anhydrous sodium carbonate in the proportion 2 ml of specimen to 50 mg of the reagent.
- If the delay before examination is to be less than 24 hours the specimens may be mixed with an equal volume of 23% trisodium phosphate solution and the time of addition of this agent to the specimen must be stated on the request form.

Transport of specimens

When specimens are sent from a clinic to a laboratory or from one laboratory to another it is important that they arrive in a satisfactory condition for the tests required and that they do not leak or offer any hazard of infection to those who transport them or handle them while in transit.

Speedy transport is essential for good results. Delays allow unwanted organisms, present in most specimens, to multiply with the result that cultures are contaminated and the organisms sought cannot be found. The fact that there are preservation methods (see above) is no reason for complacency; they are all suboptimal. Managers often seek to 'integrate' transport of pathological material with that of other material. This usually operates to the detriment of the specimens, the result of the examinations and the care of the patients.

Local transport

Many specimens are delivered by hand within hospitals or by local transport between hospitals and laboratories. Boxes of metal or thermoresistant plastic should be provided. They should be made to hold a number of specimen containers, packed vertically so that they are not likely to leak, and with each, preferably, in a separate plastic bag. These boxes should not be too large or too heavy for one person to carry as he or she may have to travel some distance. The lid should be securely fastened and in some areas it may be desirable for it to be locked. The boxes should be disinfected and then scrubbed clean at regular intervals.

Mail and air transport

Requirements and recommendations for the safe transport of pathological specimens, including cultures, are given in various national and international codes of practice and guidelines; see, for example, those published by the World Health

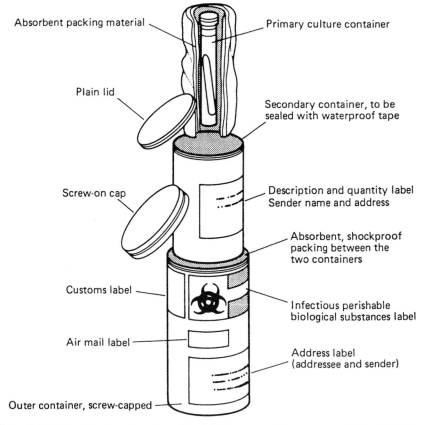

Figure 5.1 Triple packaging system for mailing infectious material as recommended by the World Health Organization (from Collins *et al.*, 1995)

Organization (1993a). The postal and transport authorities of most countries, and the International Air Transport Association, make regulations about conveying such material. All these should be consulted.

In principle, pathological material intended for postal or air transport should be in approved, robust, leak-proof, 'primary' containers which are packed into 'secondary' containers, made of metal, wood or strong cardboard, with enough absorbent material so that if they leak or are damaged the fluids will be absorbed (Figure 5.1). For sending material across international or state boundaries this container may have to be packed in the same way in an outer container and special administrative arrangements with the postal authorities and airlines may be necessary.

6

Direct smears

Direct microscopical examination of pathological material for acid-fast bacilli may be either a valuable or quite useless procedure depending on the nature and quality of the specimen. Diagnosis may be delayed, or inappropriate results obtained, if the medical staff fail to obtain suitable specimens and deliver them promptly to the laboratory with correct documentation.

Preparation of specimens

Sputum

The specimen is either spread directly on a microscope slide or concentrated by centrifugation after treatment, if necessary, to lower its specific gravity so that any mycobacteria are more easily deposited. There is evidence that concentration of bacilli in sputum by use of the cytocentrifuge increases the sensitivity of microscopy to that of culture on solid media (Saceanu *et al.*, 1993; Fodor, 1995). The microscopical examination of direct smears of sputum is probably the most useful test for the diagnosis of tuberculosis in control programmes as it permits the rapid detection of infectious patients as well as monitoring the efficacy of treatment.

The sputum specimen is examined by eye, and its appearance and consistency are recorded, e.g. as mucoid, mucopurulent, purulent, blood-stained. Further specimens should be requested if the specimen is obviously saliva.

The subsequent step of the procedure is hazardous to unskilled operators and great care is necessary to avoid contaminating the surrounding areas or releasing airborne droplets (sputum itself is, fortunately, not easily aerosolized).

The smears may be made directly from the specimen or from a centrifuged deposit after it has been digested, as described below. Sputum is not an easy material to manipulate and the normal tools of bacteriologists are usually too thin and springy to transfer the most rewarding parts of a specimen to a slide or to a tube or bottle for digestion. Very thick (2 mm diameter) nicrome wire is available but requires special loop holders. The flaming of loops may be hazardous and alcohol-sand bottles and hooded microbunsens should be used (Figure 2.6, p. 20).

The best tools for handling sputum are undoubtedly the plastic disposable loops now commercially available. The larger, 10 μl, size is the most convenient but the smaller, 1 μl, loops are useful for separating the chosen part of the specimen from the remainder. It is often necessary to use two loops for this purpose. Alternatives are throat swabs and the wooden sticks from which they are made. An advantage of all these tools is that they may be discarded into disinfectants without the need to flame them.

Although satisfactory for making direct smears, these instruments are not ideal for the preparation of centrifuged deposits as larger volumes of sputum are required: encouraging purulent or very mucoid material from its original containers into those used for processing can be a very messy and hazardous business if it is done with loops or sticks. Ordinary pipettes are unsatisfactory because sputum is too thick to be drawn in through the small holes in their tips. The most useful tools are pieces of glass tubing, about 4 mm internal diameter, cut into 200 mm lengths. One end is rounded off in a Bunsen flame to accept a rubber teat or pipetting device while the other end is left rough and sharp. The teat is compressed and the sharp end of the tubing is placed in the sputum and rotated. It will cut the sputum, allowing it to be drawn into the tube. When sufficient material has been drawn into the tube, rotating it again frees the end of the sputum and the contents may be discharged into another container.

New slides should be used whenever possible. It is not good practice to wash and re-use them, especially if they have been used for material containing acid-fast bacilli. The slides should be numbered with a diamond-pointed stylus. Grease pencil or felt-tipped pen marks are frequently washed off during staining. Pencil can be used on slides with frosted ends.

For making smears, place the slides on glass or ceramic tiles, preferably black, or on pieces of plain paper. The tiles are disinfected or the paper incinerated after each batch of slides has been prepared. In some laboratories the slides are placed on special racks or slide holders while the smears are made (Figure 2.6, p. 21). These holders should be placed on the tiles or paper. It is not good practice to spread sputum on slides resting directly on the bench or the floor of the safety cabinet.

Select a small portion of purulent or mucopurulent material, separate it from the remainder with loops or sticks and transfer it to the slide. Take care to avoid placing too much on the slide as it will not spread properly and the smear will then be too thick and may even float off the slide during staining. Spread the material carefully over an area equal to about two-thirds of the slide (Figure 6.1a) using a loop or stick. This should not be done energetically or sputum will be splashed over the surrounding area. It requires some practice to make evenly distributed smears. It is difficult, if not impossible, to see acid-fast bacilli in thick smears but thin smears may contain too few bacilli for them to be found.

Sputum should on no account be squashed between two slides. The old technique of pressing sputum between slides and drawing them apart while passing them through a Bunsen flame is particularly hazardous. Dried particles become airborne and are easily inhaled. Safety cabinets cannot be relied upon to protect workers from such dangerous practices.

Take care to avoid contamination of the fingers. Gloves, if available, should be worn. At this and all subsequent stages handle slides with forceps. Slides may be dried in the safety cabinet on racks or removed and dried on a slide drying rack by gentle heat. As soon as they are dry, fix the slides by passing them through a Bunsen flame three times or, preferably, heat them on an electric slide heater at 70–75 °C for 2 hours. Heating does not necessarily kill tubercle bacilli

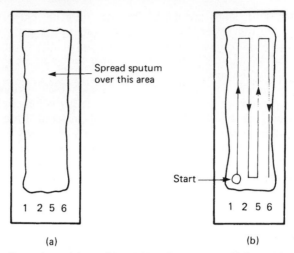

Figure 6.1 Spreading and examining a slide. (a) Spread sputum, etc. thinly over the area indicated. (b) Scan the stained smear systematically, field by field for 100–300 fields

(Allen, 1981) and the slides should still be regarded as infectious. Do not leave slides unstained or uncovered on the bench. If it is necessary to leave them for any period, place them in buffered formalin for 5 minutes and then dry them.

Buffered formalin is prepared as follows:

Formalin solution, commercial (about 37% formaldehyde)	500 ml
Sodium dihydrogen phosphate (NaH$_2$PO$_4$.H$_2$O)	22.75 g
Disodium hydrogen phosphate (Na$_2$HPO$_4$.12H$_2$O)	32.5 g
Distilled water	4.5 l

Concentrated sputum

In some laboratories direct smears are made from the centrifuged deposits after digesting and concentrating the sputum. Any of the methods of concentration described for culture (p. 61) may be used.

The procedures for making the smears are the same as those for making direct smears of sputum but as the deposit is aqueous and much less viscous there are greater hazards from aerosol production. The procedures should not under any circumstances be done on the open bench. The smears should be made with great care to avoid splashing and aerosol production and they should be thin or the material will float off during staining. Concentrated material is less adherent to slides than sputum. Care must be taken to ensure that no acid-fast bacilli are introduced during preparation or staining of the specimen. Deionized water should never be used as this is a well-known source of such bacilli and a cause of 'false' positive results (p. 56; Collins *et al.*, 1981).

Induced sputum, bronchoscopy material and transtracheal aspirates

These specimens may be processed in the same way as ordinary sputum specimens. Bulky specimens should be centrifuged before processing.

Gastric washings

Microscopical examination should be avoided as the results can be misleading. Acid-fast bacilli are frequently present in food and water and hence gain access to the stomach. There is no way of distinguishing such environmental mycobacteria from tubercle bacilli by microscopy and positive smears must be regarded with suspicion.

Laryngeal swabs

Direct smears are almost useless. Positive results are rarely encountered and negative results are meaningless. It is best to conserve what little material there is for culture.

Pus and thick aspirates

Direct smears of these materials should be very thin, as thick smears tend to float off the slides and, even if they are retained, acid-fast bacilli may be difficult to see after staining. Smears of concentrates may be prepared as for sputum. Problems may arise with either kind of smear if a large amount of blood is present in the specimen as it sometimes produces acid-fast artefacts.

Pleural fluids

Centrifuge the fluid and prepare smears from the deposit. Again, these should be thin or they may float off the slides.

Cerebrospinal fluid

Centrifuge the specimens. In cases of tuberculous meningitis there is usually very little deposit and care must be taken to conserve it. Make two parallel marks, about 10 mm long and 2 mm apart, with a diamond marker on a clean glass slide. This clearly marks the area to be searched for acid-fast bacilli. Spread a loopful of the deposit between these marks and allow it to dry. Then spread another loopful over the first and, after drying, repeat the process three or four times, depending on how much deposit is available. Some material should obviously be retained for culture. It is desirable that the smears are examined by two independent microscopists.

Some workers recommend microscopical examination of any 'spider clots' that may be present. This is difficult and we consider that such clots should be used for culture.

Urine

Avoid examination of direct smears of urine as this may give unreliable results. Environmental mycobacteria are commonly present in the lower urethra and, even with good collection techniques, their presence in specimens is unavoidable. Older accounts refer to the frequent presence of the 'smegma bacillus' (*M.*

smegmatis) in urine but this species is, in fact, rarely encountered. This term was probably used collectively for a range of saprophytic, usually scotochromogenic, mycobacteria found in urine. There is no truth in the story that tubercle bacilli and saprophytic mycobacteria can be differentiated by their relative acid- and alcohol-fastness (see p. 56). The presence of acid-fast, or acid-alcohol-fast, bacilli in direct smears of urine should therefore always be viewed with suspicion.

Faeces, blood and bone marrow

Direct smears of faeces are worthless for the diagnosis of tuberculosis as saprophytic acid-fast bacilli are frequently present in the intestine. Huge numbers of *M. avium* may, however, be detected in faeces of AIDS patients owing to extensive intestinal involvement. Smears of blood and bone marrow may likewise reveal numerous acid-fast bacilli in AIDS patients but great care must be taken in distinguishing mycobacteria from acid-fast artefacts caused by blood.

Biopsy material

Smears made from 'tubercles' or lymph nodes may reveal acid-fast bacilli, especially if scrapings are made from the inner walls of caseating lesions rather than from the caseous material itself.

Milk

Direct smears of cows' milk are of very little value, even when the milk is collected from individual teats. Other acid-fast bacilli are frequently present and cannot be distinguished microscopically from tubercle bacilli.

Staining methods

There are two standard methods of staining smears for acid-fast bacilli—The Ziehl-Nielsen (ZN) and the fluorescence microscopy (FM) techniques. The former requires an ordinary light microscope and the latter an instrument with ultraviolet illumination. Where both microscopes are available, the choice of method is influenced by the numbers of slides to be examined at any one time. The ZN is the method of choice if this number is not large, e.g. about 10 or 12, but for larger numbers much time may be saved and operator fatigue reduced by using the FM method.

In a comparative study by Kubica (1980) it was found that if the criterion for a positive FM smear was finding three fluorescent acid-fast bacilli, the method was as reliable as the ZN method. On the other hand we have noted that in several British laboratories the FM method gave more 'false positives' than the ZN procedure. We recommend, therefore, that positive FM smears should be confirmed by overstaining the smear by the ZN method.

The Ziehl-Nielsen (ZN) method

The property of acid-fastness was discovered by Paul Ehrlich in 1883, the year after the discovery of the tubercle bacillus by Robert Koch. Modifications to Ehrlich's method were subsequently made by Ziehl and Nielsen, whose names the method bears. For further details of the interesting history of this staining technique see Bishop and Neumann (1970) and Allen and Hinkes (1982). The principle of all staining techniques, including fluorescent methods, is the same. The slide is first treated with an arylmethane stain such as carbol fuchsin or a fluorescent analogue, then washed with a dilute mineral acid in water or alcohol and finally counterstained.

There are several different formulations of the carbol-fuchsin stain, the acid or acid-alcohol decolorizing mixture and the counterstain for use in the Ziehl-Nielsen (ZN) method. Some workers prefer a blue and others a green counter-stain. Colour-blind workers are advised to use a picric acid solution which gives a yellow background. In our laboratories we use a green counterstain for most specimens as this gives a soft background against which the red acid-fast bacilli are easily seen. A blue counterstain is used for films of cultures when the majority of the film is red with red acid-fast bacilli and possible contaminants will be stained blue.

Two methods for ZN staining are given here.

The traditional ZN stain

(1)	Basic fuchsin	5 g
	Phenol crystals	25 g
	Ethanol, 95%	50 ml
	Distilled water	500 ml

Dissolve the fuchsin and phenol in the ethanol over a warm water-bath and then add the water. Filter before use.

(2)	Ethanol, 95%	970 ml
	Conc. hydrochloric acid	30 ml
(3)	Malachite green	2.5 g
	OR Methylene blue	2.5 g
	OR Picric acid	3.5 g
	Distilled water	500 ml

Hold the slides bearing the smears in forceps and fix them by passing them through a Bunsen or spirit lamp flame twice in quick succession. Place them on a staining rack over a sink.

Pour freshly filtered carbol-fuchsin solution over the slides so that the smears are completely covered and heat from below with a spirit lamp flame until steam rises. Alternatively, use an electric heating plate. Leave the heated slides for 3–5 minutes. Do not allow them to dry.

Wash the slides well with running water and use forceps to turn and drain them. Return them to the rack and pour the acid-alcohol mixture over them. Allow to act for 2–3 minutes, then replace it with fresh acid-alcohol for a further 3–4 minutes.

Pour off the acid-alcohol, drain the slides and pour on the blue, green or yellow counterstain. Leave for 1–2 minutes, wash off with running water and stand the slides on edge to drain and/or blot them gently, each with a fresh piece of blotting paper, and complete the drying by heating gently over a flame.

The Tan Thiam Hok staining method
This is a 'cold' staining method (Tan Thiam Hok, 1962) which is useful in the field, when hot staining may pose difficulties.

(1)	Basic fuchsin	20 g
	Phenol crystals	40 g
	Ethanol, 95%	100 ml
	Distilled water	500 ml

Dissolve as for the ZN stain.

(2)	Methylene blue	5 g
	Ethanol, 95%	150 ml
	Distilled water	250 ml
	Sulphuric acid, 96%	100 ml

Dissolve the methylene blue in the ethanol, add the water and then the sulphuric acid, carefully and very slowly. Wear eye protection.

Fix the slides as described above, stain with the fuchsin solution for 3 minutes. Wash with tap water for 30 seconds. Flood the slides with solution (2). Leave for 1 minute, then wash as before and dry.

Fluorescent staining method

There are several variations of the basic method. Some use auramine (as below); others use a mixture of auramine and rhodamine.

(1)	Auramine	1.5 g
	Phenol crystals	15 g
	Distilled water	500 ml
(2)	Sodium chloride	3 g
	Conc. hydrochloric acid	3 ml
	Ethanol, 95%	450 ml
(3)	Potassium permanganate	0.5 g
	Distilled water	500 ml

Fix the slides as described above. Cover with the auramine-phenol solution and leave for 4 minutes. Wash off with running water and decolorize with solution (2) for a further 4 minutes. Pour this off and cover the slides with solution (3) and leave for 1 minute. Wash and dry.

Monitor the ultraviolet source used in fluorescence microscopy regularly with a Blak-ray meter. Include a positive control slide every time the microscope is used to check the staining procedure and to see if the system is working correctly.

Bulk staining methods

In bulk staining, i.e. processing a number, and succession, of slides in the same solution in a single container, there is the possibility that acid-fast bacilli might float off one slide and become attached to others, giving 'false positive' results. Many bacteriologists have therefore counselled against this method.

On the other hand, it can save a great deal of time and materials. Clancy *et al.* (1976) found no false positives when they used the Shandon-Elliot automatic staining machine for processing large numbers of slides by the FM method. Fodor (1984) rinsed, decolorized and counterstained carbol-fuchsin stained smears in common containers without encountering false positives.

Quantitative microscopy

The numbers of acid-fast bacilli vary considerably in sputum samples taken, even at close intervals of time, from the same patient. Thus, quantitative microscopy gives a rather crude indication of the severity of disease, the degree of infectivity and the response to therapy. Nevertheless, some physicians request a quantitative result which is achieved by scanning at least 100 microscope fields of ZN stained smears as indicated in Figure 6.1b (p. 50) and counting the number of bacilli seen. At least 300 fields should be examined, however, before the smear is reported negative. Table 6.1 shows a reporting system in common use.

Reporting direct smears

It should not be assumed that acid-fast bacilli are tubercle bacilli. It is best and safest merely to report that acid-fast bacilli were seen in the direct smear.

'False positive' smears

There are several reasons for 'false positive' findings in direct smears. Slides that have been used before may retain acid-fast bacilli and scratches on old slides may retain the fuchsin and look like acid-fast bacilli. The possibility of

Table 6.1 Quantitative microscopy of direct sputum smears

No. of bacilli seen	Report
None in 300 fields	Negative
1–2 in 300 fields	Doubtful; repeat
1–10 in 100 fields	+
1–10 in 10 fields	++
1–10 in 1 field	+++
> 10 in 1 field	++++

This is a logarithmic scale which facilitates plotting

acid-fast bacilli floating off one slide and attaching to others during bulk staining is discussed above. Blotting paper, if used for drying several slides in succession, may carry over acid-fast bacilli.

Water used to prepare staining solutions may become contaminated by environmental mycobacteria. This is more likely to occur if deionized water is used as such bacilli may colonize deionizer resin and the tubing connecting the deionizer to the tap. Such contamination may result in 'outbreaks' of false positive results. A sudden increase in the number of positive slides, or a series of consecutive positives, should arouse suspicion but may only be revealed by examination of the laboratory records. Two incidents where acid-fast and fluorescent artefacts were found in water, one from a storage tank and one from demineralized water, were reported by Collins *et al.* (1981).

Positive smears—negative cultures

It can be embarrassing if a laboratory reports that acid-fast bacilli were seen in a direct smear but fails to grow mycobacteria from the same specimen. There are several explanations. One is that the staining solutions are contaminated by acid-fast bacilli or artefacts, as described above. Another is that technical and clerical errors occurred during microscopy and documentation. There may also be non-technical reasons. The specimen may contain psychrophilic mycobacteria that fail to grow at the incubation temperature. Sputum which is smear-positive and culture-negative is occasionally obtained from patients with advanced cavitating disease and from patients who have received anti-tuberculosis drugs (Dominguez and Vivas, 1977; Taik Chae Kim *et al.*, 1984): the acid-fast bacilli are dead.

'Acid and alcohol-fast bacilli'

There is no basis for the old story that tubercle bacilli are acid- and alcohol-fast while other mycobacteria are only acid-fast. Acid-fastness varies with the physiological state of the organisms. The alcohol in the decolorizing solution merely gives a cleaner stained smear.

Storage and disposal of slides

Slides of positive smears should be retained for several weeks and until the cultures are positive, in case the results are questioned. Immersion oil may be removed with toluene or xylene and the slides stored in commercially available slide boxes that have tightly fitting lids.

Negative slides should also be kept until the cultures are discarded as negative.

7
Cultural methods

The usual microbiological techniques of plating clinical material on selective or enrichment media and subculturing to obtain pure cultures cannot be applied to tuberculosis bacteriology. Most pathogenic mycobacteria grow slowly, taking two to six weeks, or even longer, to give visible growth. Special media and techniques not used for other organisms are required. Cultures are usually made in tubes or bottles rather than in Petri dishes because mycobacteria, especially tubercle bacilli, are present in very small numbers in most specimens. This necessitates comparatively large inocula which are spread evenly over the surface of the medium. The bottles are tightly stoppered to prevent drying of the medium, which would certainly happen in Petri dishes. Moreover, opening Petri dish cultures is more likely to release aerosols than opening bottles or tubes.

Culture media

Many different culture media have been devised for growing the tubercle bacillus and other mycobacteria but relatively few of them are in use today. Those currently used are egg-based and agar-based solid media and liquid media.

For the culture of sputum the egg-based media are the first choice. There is evidence, however, that liquid media, especially those containing antibiotic mixtures, give better results with other specimens (Allen *et al.*, 1983; Mitchison *et al.*, 1983). Both kinds of media should be used for specimens that are non-repeatable, e.g. biopsy material or cerebrospinal fluid. We consider that both egg-based and liquid media should also be used for culturing urine deposits.

Egg-based media

The most popular of these are the various modifications of Löwenstein-Jensen medium. Others include Ogawa and Stonebrink medium and those of the American Thoracic Society (ATS) and the International Union Against Tuberculosis (IUAT). We prefer Löwenstein-Jensen medium and in this book the initials LJG are used for medium containing glycerol and LJP for that containing pyruvate. The former supports growth of *M. tuberculosis* and the latter *M. bovis*, most strains of which cannot utilize glycerol as a carbon source. Both should be used in regions where patients might be infected with either organism. Some other mycobacteria, e.g. the *M. avium* complex and *M. malmoense*, also grow better on LJP. Löwenstein-Jensen media, in tubes or bottles and ready for use, are commercially available in some countries.

Löwenstein-Jensen medium

There are several variations. Some contain asparagine and/or potato starch but neither are necessary and the medium described below does not contain them. All containers and other equipment must be sterilized before use as the process of inspissation (coagulation) will not kill all contaminating micro-organisms, especially not spores.

Monopotassium phosphate (KH_2PO_4), anhydrous	4.0 g
Magnesium sulphate ($MgSO_4.7H_2O$)	0.4 g
Magnesium citrate	1.0 g
Glycerol (analytical grade), for LJG only	20 ml
OR sodium pyruvate, for LJP only	12.0 g
Distilled water, to	1000 ml
Whole fresh eggs	1600 ml
Malachite green, 1% w/v aqueous solution	50 ml

Dissolve the salts and glycerol in the distilled water and steam in autoclave or steamer at atmospheric pressure for 2 hours. This is the mineral salt solution which may be prepared in bulk and stored. Wash the eggs with soap and water, rinse in 70% alcohol and wipe dry. Break the eggs into a screw-capped jar containing a few large (c. 10 mm diameter) glass beads and shake to break the yolks and to homogenize the material. Alternatively use a sterilizable homogenizer such as a Waring blender, if available. Filter through sterile gauze into a graduated cylinder until the 1600 ml mark is reached and add to the mineral salt solution. Add the malachite green solution and mix well. (As a further precaution against contamination, 200 000 units of penicillin may also be added.) Dispense as required, e.g. in 7 ml amounts in 28 ml screw-capped bottles. Place the bottles on sloped racks and inspissate at 80–85 °C until the medium is hard. This takes around 50–90 minutes; the actual time required depends on the thickness of the glass of the bottles and the temperature of the oven. An oven fitted with a fan is preferable as this ensures that the bottles are heated evenly.

Acid egg medium (Zaher and Marks, 1977)

This may be used to avoid neutralization and centrifugation of the sputum homogenate decontaminated by use of NaOH (see below). It is commercially available in some countries.

Monopotassium phosphate (KH_2PO_4), anhydrous	6.3 g
Magnesium sulphate ($MgSO_4.7H_2O$)	0.3 g
Glycerol (analytical grade)	12 ml
OR sodium pyruvate	7.0 g
N hydrochloric acid	32 ml
Distilled water, to	600 ml
Whole fresh eggs (prepared as for LJ, see above)	1100 ml

Malachite green, 1% w/v aqueous solution   22 ml
Penicillin, sodium salt   100 000 units
Prepare as for LJ medium (see above).

Agar-based media

Although several agar-based media have been proposed for the culture of
mycobacteria, only Middlebrook's 7H10 medium (Middlebrook and Cohn,
1958) and its modification, 7H11 (Cohn *et al.*, 1968), are in general use today in
diagnostic laboratories. They are complex media and it is best to purchase them
as dehydrated powders. They require the addition of an oleic acid-albumin-
dextrose-catalase (OADC) supplement, commercially available in the liquid
form. These media may not be as successful as egg-based media for primary
isolation but they are more convenient in areas where egg-based media cannot
been made or are too bulky to import.

The antibiotic mixture of Mitchison *et al.* (1972, 1983) may be added (per
litre): polymyxin B, 200 000 units; carbenicillin, 50 mg; trimethoprim, 10 mg;
amphotericin, 10 mg.

Liquid media

Kirchner medium allows relatively large inocula to be used, e.g. for cerebrospinal, pericardial, pleural or peritoneal fluids and specimens expected to
contain very few mycobacteria. The addition of the Mitchison antibiotic mixture
(see above) may avoid the necessity for decontaminating the specimens.

Kirchner medium

Disodium phosphate (Na2HPO$_4$.12H$_2$O)   19.0 g
Asparagine   5.0 g
Monopotassium phosphate (KH$_2$PO$_4$), anhydrous   2.5 g
Trisodium citrate   2.5 g
Magnesium sulphate (MgSO$_4$.7H$_2$O)   0.6 g
Glycerol   20.0 ml
Phenol red, 0.4% w/v aqueous solution   3.0 ml
Distilled water   to 1000 ml

Steam to dissolve. Adjust pH, if necessary, to 7.4–7.6. Dispense in 9 ml
amounts in 25 ml screw-capped bottles and autoclave at 115 °C for 10 minutes.
When cool add 1 ml of sterile horse serum (or Middlebrook OADC enrichment
if indicated) to each bottle. The antibiotic mixture of Mitchison (see above) may
be added.

Large amounts of fluid, e.g. pericardial, pleural or peritoneal, may be added
directly (at the bedside) to equal quantities of double-strength Kirchner medium.

Middlebrook 7H9 broth

This medium is a complex one and it is best to purchase it as a dehydrated
powder. It is used in several identification tests as well as for primary isolation.
Related broths, e.g. 7H12B and 7H13A, are commercially available for use in
radiometric systems (p. 67).

Pretreatment of specimens

Most material submitted for culture contains many micro-organisms which grow rapidly and would thus soon overgrow the entire surface of the medium and probably digest it before mycobacteria started to grow. Growth of these organisms may be suppressed by the use of an 'antibiotic cocktail', such as that of Mitchison, described above. There are, however, no antibiotics or dyes, singly or in combinations, that can be totally relied on to suppress the growth of certain organisms (e.g. pseudomonads and fungi) that may be present in pathological material.

Specimens known to contain other organisms must be treated in an attempt to destroy them but preserve the mycobacteria. The reagents used must also reduce the viscosity of the specimen so that it can be centrifuged with a reasonable certainty that the majority of the mycobacteria will be deposited. Unfortunately, there are no reagents that will completely fulfil the first requirement and tuberculosis bacteriologists have learnt to steer a middle course and to accept that if enough mycobacteria to give a diagnosis are to survive then a proportion of cultures will be contaminated with 'resistant' organisms such as *Pseudomonas aeruginosa*, some enterobacteria and streptococci, and a range of yeasts and microfungi. Experience has shown that a contamination rate of 2–3% is acceptable in laboratories that receive freshly obtained specimens. If, on the other hand, specimens, especially sputum, take several days to reach the laboratory, or cannot be processed immediately, then the contamination rate may be as high as 10%. Refrigeration of specimens does not markedly reduce the contamination rate. It may be argued that a laboratory which experiences no contaminated cultures is probably using a method that kills many mycobacteria.

Although many chemicals have been investigated, comparatively few have proved to be reasonably successful. Those known to be satisfactory are divided into two groups as described below.

(1) 'Soft' reagents that have a minimal effect on both mycobacteria and the other organisms (which are usually termed 'contaminants'). These reagents are suitable for fresh specimens that can be processed immediately, i.e. when the number of contaminants is small and they have not had the opportunity to multiply. The time of exposure to the reagents is not critical.
(2) 'Hard' reagents which will kill mycobacteria as well as other organisms unless exposure time is carefully controlled. They are very effective against most contaminants.

After treatment, a centrifuged deposit is usually seeded on culture media but, in two of the methods described below, uncentrifuged material may be used. Although these methods are not optimal, they avoid the hazards of centrifugation (see p. 28) and reduce the time required for processing large numbers of specimens.

All manipulations should be conducted in a microbiological safety cabinet. Sealed buckets should be used for centrifugation and the centrifuge operated at 2000–3000 g. Use of centrifuges operating at less than 2000 g give no better results than methods not employing centrifugation.

It is better to dispense reagents in measured volumes in screw-capped bottles, one bottle per specimen, and to sterilize them ready for use. Pipetting reagents from stock bottles during the procedure, or using 'squeezy bottles', may lead to cross contamination.

Sputum

Avoid pooling sputum specimens as it frequently distributes contaminants. Large amounts, e.g. more than 5 ml, also cause problems. For advice on manipulating sputum see p. 48.

Trisodium phosphate method

Use this 'soft' method for fresh specimens of sputum, gastric aspirates, bronchoscopy material and other specimens that are not likely to be heavily contaminated with other organisms.

Add about 2 ml of sputum to a bottle containing 3 ml of 23% w/v trisodium phosphate ($Na_3PO_4.12H_2O$) solution. Blend for 2 minutes on a vortex mixer. Allow the mixture to stand at room temperature for 12–18 hours. Add 16 ml of sterile distilled water, centrifuge for 20 minutes at 2000–3000 g and inoculate the deposit on to suitable media.

Sodium hydroxide method

This is a 'hard' method and is suitable for material that is likely to be heavily contaminated.

Add about 1 ml of sputum to a bottle containing 2 ml of 1N (4% w/v) NaOH in a screw-cap tube. Mix well on a vortex mixer, allow to stand for 15 minutes (thin specimens) or not more than 30 minutes (thick specimens) with occasional shaking. (Incubation at 37 °C has not been shown to hasten digestion; nor has mechanical shaking (Collins, 1951).) Neutralize by adding the contents of one bottle (3 ml) of 14% w/v solution of monopotassium phosphate (KH_2PO_4; anhydrous) containing enough phenol red indicator, around 40 mg/l, to impart a yellow colour (this turns red when neutralization is complete). Centrifuge for 20 minutes at 2000–3000 g and inoculate the deposit on suitable media.

Oxalic acid method

This is a very 'hard' method but is particularly useful if the specimen is likely to contain *Pseudomonas* species; e.g. sputum from patients with cystic fibrosis.

Add about 1 ml of sputum to a bottle containing 3 ml of 3% oxalic acid. Blend for 2 minutes on a vortex mixer and allow to stand for 10–15 minutes. Add 16 ml of sterile distilled water and centrifuge as described above. Culture the deposit.

Methods avoiding centrifugation

(1) Add not more than 1 ml of homogenate treated with either trisodium phosphate or sodium hydroxide after dilution or neutralization to a tube of Kirchner medium.

(2) Mycobacteria may be concentrated by a flocculation technique. Add a few drops of a mixture of 1.5% w/v calcium chloride ($CaCl_2.2H_2O$) and 1.5% barium chloride ($BaCl_2.2H_2O$), mixed immediately before use, to 10 ml of the

sputum/trisodium phosphate mixture and stand overnight. Remove the flocculated sediment with a pipette and inoculate the media.

(3) Inoculate a tube of acid egg medium (p. 58) with exactly 0.2 ml (the amount is critical) of material treated with 4% sodium hydroxide and incubate.

Laryngeal swabs

Add enough oxalic acid to cover the swab in its original tube. Allow to act for 15 minutes. Remove the swab to another tube containing sterile distilled water to dilute the acid. After a few minutes lift the swab, allow it to drain and inoculate culture media.

In addition, for optimal results, transfer the oxalic acid, which may contain tubercle bacilli washed off the swab, to another tube and centrifuge it. Wash the deposit with distilled water, centrifuge again and inoculate media with the deposit.

Urine

Centrifuge about 25 ml of urine, preferably an early morning specimen, at 3000 g for 20 minutes. Examine a Gram-stained smear of the deposit and assess the number of non-acid-fast bacteria, or inoculate blood agar and incubate it overnight, meanwhile refrigerating the remainder of the deposit.

Suspend the deposit in 2 ml of 4% sulphuric acid and allow to stand for 15 to 40 minutes, depending on the number of non-acid-fast organisms present. Dilute with 15 ml of sterile distilled water and centrifuge again. Culture the deposit.

Pleural, cerebrospinal and other fluids

Assess the number of non-acid-fast organisms as for urines. If there are none, culture the centrifuged deposit without further treatment. Break up clots or cut them with sterile scissors.

If other organisms are present, mix the deposit with 2 ml of 4% sulphuric acid and allow to stand for 15 to 40 minutes, depending on the number of non-acid-fast organisms present. Dilute with 15 ml of sterile distilled water and centrifuge again. Culture the deposit.

In addition, as mycobacteria in the fluids (especially in the case of cerebrospinal fluids) may adhere to glass or plastic surfaces, add one of the liquid media containing antibiotics to the original container.

Large amounts of fluid, e.g. pleural or pericardial fluid, may be added directly to an equal volume of double strength Kirchner medium at the bedside.

Pus

Treat this in the same way as aspirated fluids, but if any non-acid-fast organisms are present or if the material is very thick, treat in the same way as sputum.

Blood and bone marrow

Add 8.5 ml of blood to 1.5 ml of 0.35% sodium polyethanolium sulphate (SPS; the anticoagulant least toxic to mycobacteria). Mix well and add 1 ml volumes to 10–20 ml volumes of Middlebrook 7H9 medium containing 0.025% SPS and the antibiotic mixture of Mitchison (p. 59). Add 1 ml amounts of bone marrow directly to the Middlebrook medium.

The isolator-10 lysis centrifugation system (Du Pont) is useful (Kiehn and Cammarata, 1988). Collect 10 ml of blood into the tubes which contain anti-coagulant and saponin which lyses the blood. Centrifuge for 30 minutes and culture the deposit.

Blood and bone marrow may be inoculated directly into Bactec 13B medium for radiometric detection of mycobacterial growth. The bottles are under vacuum to accept up to 5 ml of the specimen. The enrichment, 0.5 ml, supplied with the medium, is then added and the bottles incubated in the Bactec system at 37 °C (see p. 67).

Faeces

Suspend about 1 g of faeces in sterile distilled water and allow to stand for 1–2 minutes. Remove the supernatant material and treat it as for sputum by the sodium hydroxide method and culture the deposit on or in medium containing the Mitchison antibiotic mixture.

Tissue

Cut lymph nodes and other tissues into small pieces, using a sterile scalpel or scissors, and then homogenize in a Griffith tube or a mechanical blender. Assess the numbers of non-acid-fast bacilli as described above and then treat as for fluids or pus.

Milk

Centrifuge at least 100 ml of milk. Treat separately the cream layer and the de-posit by the sodium hydroxide or oxalic acid methods and culture the deposits.

Water

(1) Filter at least 2 litres of water through a membrane filter. Aseptically remove the membrane from the filter, cut it into strips not more than 1 cm wide and place each strip in 3% oxalic acid in a Petri dish for 15 minutes. Remove to distilled water for 5 minutes and then place each strip on the surface of media in screw-capped bottles. Alternatively place the membrane filter in Kirchner medium containing antibiotics.

(2) Add cetyl pyridinium chloride to the water to give a final concentration of 2% and stand for 12–18 hours. Centrifuge and inoculate the required media or filter and place the membrane in Kirchner medium as above.

Inoculation of culture media

A common fault is the use of too small an inoculum. Use a plastic Pasteur pipette, rather than a loop, to inoculate each slope with 0.2 to 0.4 ml of the centrifuged deposit. Fluid media can accommodate up to 1 ml of inoculum.

Inoculate at least two slopes of egg medium, one LJG and the other LJP. Place the slopes in a horizontal position for an hour or two after they have been inoculated to allow the inoculum to be absorbed. Otherwise, most of it runs to the bottom of the tube and may never be in contact with the medium.

If possible, retain some of the inoculum, especially of non-repeatable specimens, refrigerated at −20 °C.

Incubation

Incubate cultures at 35–37 °C. In addition, incubate duplicate cultures of material from superficial lesions at 30–33 °C. Incubate cultures on solid medium in a vertical position so that individual colonies may develop. If the incubator is fitted with an internal light to facilitate the early recognition of photochromogens, the surfaces of the culture media should face the light source. Strains of *M. bovis* grow best at a slightly reduced oxygen tension. Ensure therefore that the caps of the culture tubes are tightly closed so that, as oxygen is consumed, the atmosphere becomes microaerophilic. Carbon dioxide enhances mycobacterial growth. Thus, if a suitable incubator is available, culture tubes may be incubated with the caps loosened for one week in an atmosphere of 10% carbon dioxide in air. After one week, the caps should be tightened to prevent desiccation of the medium.

Examination of cultures

Examine all cultures after 3 days and remove any that show growth for further examination. Colonies of contaminants and some rapidly growing mycobacteria may appear at this time. Thereafter, examine the cultures weekly for at least six weeks and, if possible, for eight or even 12 weeks. Some mycobacteria grow very slowly and extended incubation may thus result in a small increment of positive cultures, especially from resected material.

Discard any cultures showing obvious contamination, e.g. growth of moulds, and also those in which the medium has liquefied or turned a dark green. The latter is due to growth of micro-organisms that produce acid from constituents of the medium with a consequent lowering of the pH which unbinds some of the malachite green from the egg. Tubercle bacilli will not grow under these conditions.

Remove for further examination any cultures that show confluent growth or isolated colonies of a buff, yellow or orange colour. Close inspection, preferably with a hand lens and under a good bench lamp, is necessary to reveal very small colonies or the effuse growth which is characteristic of some environmental mycobacteria.

In Kirchner medium tubercle bacilli grow as fluffy spherical colonies, 1–2 mm in diameter, at the bottom of the tube. Shake the bottle gently to observe them and remove them with a plastic Pasteur pipette for microscopic examination and subculture on solid media. It may be difficult to recognize the smoother growth of some other mycobacteria. Examine any sediment by ZN staining.

Microscopic examination

Examine ZN-stained films of all suspicious growths. The fluorescent method fails to reveal the cellular morphology which is a helpful diagnostic criterion. It also fails to reveal the presence of non-acid-fast organisms.

Three or, with experience, four films may be made on one 76 × 25 mm slide. When large numbers of films are to be made, it is worthwhile purchasing the larger, 76 × 51 mm, slides which will accommodate up to eight.

Mark the culture numbers on the slide with a diamond stylus. Place a small drop (e.g. 10 μl) of a saturated solution of mercuric chloride near the number. This chemical kills, almost instantly, any mycobacteria that might be splashed or aerosolized during the preparation of the smear.

Remove a very small amount of growth from the culture with a loop (the 1 μl plastic loops are ideal) or a swab stick, and gently rub it into the mercuric chloride solution. Violent action may disturb the arrangement of the bacilli (see below). Note the ease with which the organisms emulsify in the liquid. Tubercle bacilli, for example, do not form smooth suspensions, unlike some other mycobacteria.

Allow the films to dry, fix in heat and stain by the ZN method. It is usually unnecessary to heat the carbol fuchsin when smears of mycobacterial cultures (as distinct from sputum, etc.) are being stained.

Figures 7.1–7.4 show the microscopical appearance of several species of mycobacteria. The arrangement of cells varies from the 'serpentine cords' usually, but not always, characteristic of tubercle bacilli, to a uniform distribution of cells. Cellular morphology is also variable, with individual bacilli ranging in length from 1 to 10 μm and in width from 0.5 to 1.5 μm. Some mycobacteria appear to be almost coccoid and others filamentous. Staining may be regular or the cells may have a beaded or banded appearance. Weakly acid-fast bacilli may also be seen: parts of the organisms stain blue or green or there may be a mixture of acid-fast and non-acid-fast bacilli. Take care with these: they may be pure cultures or a mixture of mycobacteria and other organisms (contaminants).

Preliminary identification

At this stage an experienced worker can usually say whether an acid-fast organism is likely to be a tubercle bacillus or one of the other species of mycobacteria. Tubercle bacilli do not give visible growth in primary cultures in less than one week and colonies usually take two or three weeks to appear. The colonies are buff (off-white) coloured, never yellow; they are rough, often having the appearance of breadcrumbs or cauliflowers; they do not emulsify in the fluid used for making smears but give a granular suspension. Microscopically, they may be arranged in serpentine cords (Figure 7.1), or show linear clumping; individual cells are rarely shorter than 3 μm or longer than 4 μm.

Other mycobacteria may show one or more of the following characteristics: growth appears within one week on subculture; colonies are of a yellow or orange colour; colonies emulsify readily in the fluid used for making smears;

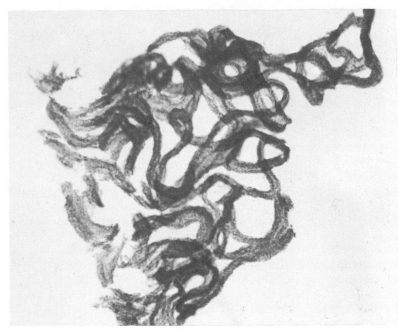

Figure 7.1 Microscopical appearance of *Mycobacterium tuberculosis*, showing serpentine cords

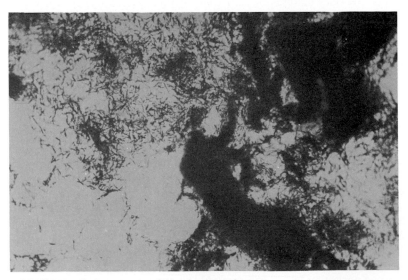

Figure 7.2 Microscopical appearance of *Mycobacterium kansasii*

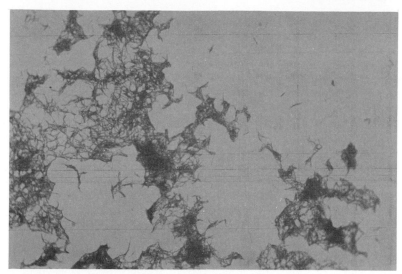

Figure 7.3 Microscopical appearance of *Mycobacterium xenopi*

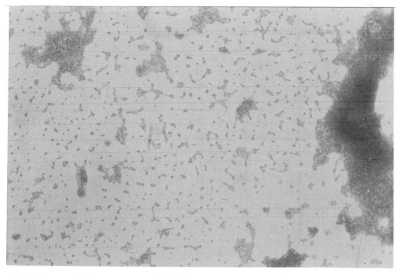

Figure 7.4 Microscopical appearance of *Mycobacterium avium* complex

cells may be less than 2 μm or more than 5 μm in length and have the microscopical appearance of those shown in Figures 7.2–7.4.

Radiometric method for mycobacterial culture

A commercial instrument (Bactec, Becton Dickinson) has been developed for the early detection of growth of mycobacteria by a radiometric method.

Sputum or other homogenates, decontaminated if necessary, are added, by injection through a rubber cap, into a vial of Middlebrook 12B medium containing antibiotics and ^{14}C-labelled palmitic acid. If growth occurs, radioactive carbon dioxide is liberated. The air space above the medium in each bottle is sampled automatically at fixed intervals and the amount of radioactive carbon dioxide is estimated and recorded.

Radiometry is not more sensitive than conventional culture methods but the readings are automated. Growth of tubercle bacilli and many other mycobacteria is usually detectable in 2 to 12 days. By transferring growth to a bottle incorporating a specific inhibitor of the growth of tubercle bacilli, p-nitro-α-acetylamino-β-hydroxypropiophenone (NAP) in the medium and also to a control bottle, it is possible to distinguish this group from other mycobacteria with an accuracy of 97–98%. Mycobacteria growing in the NAP medium are subcultured and identified by traditional methods or by nucleic acid probes.

Experience indicates that radiometry is successful and reliable and that the cost of the equipment and media can be offset by the cost-effectiveness of rapid diagnosis. The major problem with this system is the disposal of radioactive waste. Rapid non-radiometric systems have recently been developed. These include the MB BacT system (Organon Teknika) in which released carbon dioxide causes a dye in the base of the culture tube to change from green to yellow, and the MGIT (Mycobacteria Growth Indicator Tube, Becton Dickinson) which has an oxygen-quenched fluorescent dye in the bottom of the tube. Replicating mycobacteria consume oxygen dissolved in the medium, the quenching ceases and the dye fluoresces when exposed to a UV light source. These non-radiometric culture systems may be read manually or automatically. Comparative studies of the radiometric and non-radiometric systems in respect to sensitivity and rapidity are in progress.

Other culture techniques

A biphasic system (Septi-Chek AFB, Becton Dickinson) consists of a bottle of Middlebrook 7H9 liquid medium attached to a tube containing strips of Middlebrook agar and modified egg media to provide colonies for further testing and chocolate agar to detect contaminants. Detection is not so rapid as with the radiometric system but it is more rapid than with conventional culture (Salfinger *et al.*, 1990). It is suitable for laboratories that do not receive enough specimens to justify purchase of the more sophisticated systems.

Negative cultures from positive direct smear specimens

This problem is discussed on p. 56.

8

Identification of species

Most of the species of mycobacteria commonly encountered in medical and veterinary bacteriology laboratories are included in the Approved List of Bacterial Names of the International Committee on Systematic Bacteriology (Skerman *et al.*, 1980; Table 1.1, p. 2). These, and more recently described species, causing human and animal disease are listed according to the type of disease that they usually cause in Table 8.1.

Nomenclature

The tubercle bacilli

The term 'tubercle bacillus' should now be restricted to members of the *Mycobacterium tuberculosis* complex which contains four of the species in the approved lists (Skerman *et al.*, 1980); namely, *Mycobacterium tuberculosis*, *M. bovis*, *M. africanum* and the rarely encountered *M. microti*. It also contains the vaccine strain Bacille Calmette-Guérin (BCG). The terms 'avian tubercle bacillus' (*M. avium*) and 'cold-blooded tubercle bacillus' (*M. chelonae* and *M. fortuitum*) are no longer permissible.

From a clinical point of view—and here we are mainly concerned with diagnostic mycobacteriology—it is desirable, though not essential, to identify species within the *M. tuberculosis* complex.

For epidemiological purposes, however, it may be desirable to identify not only the species but also the geographical variants (classical and Asian) of *M. tuberculosis* and the two geographical variants of *M. africanum* (Collins *et al.*, 1982). Further subdivision of these variants is achievable by the use of DNA fingerprinting as described in Chapter 10.

Other species

Again, for clinical purposes, it is usually sufficient to identify the commoner species of opportunistic pathogens and to differentiate them from those mycobacteria that are unlikely to be of clinical significance but which often occur as 'contaminants' in cultures of clinical materials. There is, however, no clear distinction between opportunist pathogens and harmless saprophytes. It must be

Table 8.1 The usual causes of mycobacterial disease in humans and animals. Uncommon causes are in parentheses

(A) Disease in humans

Tuberculosis	*M. tuberculosis* (*M. bovis*, *M. africanum*)
Leprosy	*M. leprae*
Swimming-pool granuloma	*M. marinum*
Buruli ulcer	*M. ulcerans*
Post-traumatic abscesses	*M. chelonae*, *M. fortuitum* (*M. terrae*, *M. flavescens*)
Other skin lesions	(*M. haemophilum*, *M. kansasii*, *M. shinshuense*)
Lymphadenitis (usually in children)	*M. avium* complex, *M. scrofulaceum* (many other species)
Opportunist pulmonary disease	*M. avium* complex, *M. kansasii*, *M. xenopi*, *M. malmoense*, *M. scrofulaceum* (*M. asiaticum*, *M. celatum*, *M. gordonae*, *M. simiae*, *M. szulgai*, *M. chelonae*, *M. fortuitum*)
HIV-associated disseminated disease	*M. avium* complex (*M. genevense*)
Non-HIV-associated disseminated disease	*M. avium* complex, *M. chelonae*

(B) Disease in animals

Mammalian tuberculosis	*M. bovis* (*M. tuberculosis*, *M. microti*)
Avian tuberculosis	*M. avium* (*M. sylvaticum* in wood pigeons)
Lymphadenitis in pigs	*M. avium*
Lymphadenitis in deer	*M. avium*, *M. bovis*
Paratuberculosis (Johne's disease)	*M. paratuberculosis*
Farcy	*M. farcinogenes*, *M. senegalense*
Rat (and cat) 'leprosy'	*M. lepraemurium*

assumed that any mycobacterium, under given circumstances, is able to cause disease.

Identification of members of the *Mycobacterium tuberculosis* complex

Although preliminary examination of the cultures may suggest that the organisms are members of this complex, it is best to do confirmatory tests. Unfortunately, there is no completely reliable single test that will differentiate *M. tuberculosis*, *M. bovis* and *M. africanum* from all other mycobacteria. Tests that have been used are rate of growth and pigmentation (Timpe and Runyon, 1954); growth at temperatures other than 37 °C (Runyon, 1959; Marks and Trollope, 1960), inhibition by *p*-nitrobenzoic acid (PNB) (Tsukamura and Tsukamura, 1964), hydroxylamine (Tsukamura, 1970; Collins and Yates, 1979) and by *p*-nitro-acetylamino-hydroxypropiophenone (NAP) (Eidus *et al.*, 1960). The use of nucleic acid probes for this purpose is described in Chapter 10. (Some laboratory workers still use the niacin test but this has been shown to have limitations.)

The screening method of Marks (1972, 1976) has been used successfully by the Reference and Regional Tuberculosis Laboratories in England and Wales for a number of years. This screening method is adequate for clinical purposes but does not permit differentiation of the complex into the various species and their variants. The screening tests and methods for the identification of members of the *M. tuberculosis* complex are described below.

Preparation of suspensions

Suspension bottles
Wash small iron nails, or pieces of stout stainless steel wire, about 10 mm length, in ether (or first in acetone and then in ether) to remove grease. Wash glass beads, 3 mm in diameter, in weak (approx. 0.5%) hydrochloric acid to remove soda. Place one nail and 10–20 glass beads in a small screw-capped bottle containing 1 ml of phosphate buffer pH 7.4 (anhydrous disodium hydrogen phosphate (Na_2HPO_4) 6.6 g and potassium dihydrogen phosphate (KH_2PO_4) 1.75 g in 1 litre of distilled water) or prepare buffer from commercially available tablets ('Dulbecco A' phosphate buffered saline). Sterilize by autoclaving.

Preparation of bacterial suspensions
Transfer growth from the primary culture into a suspension bottle by using either a 10 μl loop or a cotton wool swab. Place the bottle on a magnetic stirrer so that the iron nail and the glass beads break up the clumps of bacteria. Stand for 5 minutes to allow the larger residual clumps of bacteria to settle. This suspension contains approximately 10^5 colony forming units/ml. Alternatively, place the bottle on a vortex mixer for about 10 seconds, but allow to stand for longer, 10 to 15 minutes, as more aerosol is generated by this technique.

Inoculation of the test media
Place the suspension bottle at an angle on modelling clay. Media are either inoculated by means of a pipette delivering 10 μl of suspension or by use of a bacteriological loop. Disposable plastic loops are preferred. Withdraw loops from the suspension edgewise so that large convex drops are not transferred.

Inoculate each of two tubes of LJG medium (and one of LJP if primary growth on this is better than on LJG) and one of PNB medium (LJG containing 500 mg/l of *p*-nitrobenzoic acid) with approximately 10 μl of the suspension. The inoculum should not be spread over the surface of the medium but streaked down the middle. This facilitates early examination as the border between growth and medium is more easily observed.

Incubation
Incubate one LJG tube and the PNB tube at 37 °C in an internally illuminated incubator. Incubate the other LJG tube at 25 ± 0.5 °C (room temperature is too variable).

If the 37 °C incubator is of the 'walk-in' type, leave the light on all the time and slope the racks of tubes so that the whole surface of the medium is illuminated. If a cabinet incubator is used it may be adapted by fitting a 6 W fluorescent lamp inside. The very small amount of heat given out by this will not affect the thermostat setting. Alternatively, incubate the slopes in the dark until growth is evident and then place them facing daylight, but not direct sunlight, on a windowsill, or facing and about 100 cm away from a tungsten filament bench lamp. After illumination for one hour, return the tubes to the incubator. Loosening the caps to admit oxygen is said to enhance pigment production.

Incubation at 25 °C may present problems, especially in centrally heated laboratories and warm climates. Incubators fitted with refrigerated coils are available and we have found them reliable. Refrigerated water-baths are not suitable for this work, even if the water level is constant: there is always the possibility that a tube may break or leak and that the water will become infected with tubercle bacilli. If the ambient temperature is below 25 °C, heated incubator blocks may be used.

Reading results

Examine the tubes after 3, 7, 14 and 21 days' incubation. Members of the *M. tuberculosis* complex require about 7 to 10 days to give visible colonies; they do not produce pigment; they do not grow at 25 °C nor do they grow on the PNB medium. At 21 days, strains of *M. tuberculosis* will show characteristic, dry, breadcrumb or cauliflower-like colonies that are greyish white or buff in colour on the 37 °C LJG and LJP medium only. There will be no growth on the PNB medium or at 25 °C. Growth of *M. bovis* and *M. africanum* is usually poor on LJG but quite good on LJP medium. The colonies are flatter and may not appear to be as rough as those of *M. tuberculosis*. Occasional strains of *M. bovis* may show very poor growth on PNB and even at 25 °C and these require further identification as described below.

Mycobacteria that grow within three days, produce yellow, orange or pink pigmented colonies, grow at 25 °C or on PNB medium, or show any combination of these characteristics are not tubercle bacilli and should be identified by the methods described below (p. 77).

Identification of species and variants of the *M. tuberculosis* complex

Make suspensions, as described above, of organisms identified as members of this complex.

Susceptibility to thiophen-2-carboxylic acid hydrazine (TCH)

Prepare LJG medium containing 5 mg/l of TCH and tube in 2 ml amounts in small screw-capped bottles. Inoculate and incubate for 2–3 weeks at 37 °C. Compare the growth with that on LJG control tubes.

According to Harrington and Karlson (1966), *M. tuberculosis* is resistant and *M. bovis* is susceptible to this compound at comparable concentrations. Yates and Collins (1979) confirmed this but found that many strains of *M. tuberculosis* from Asians were also susceptible, as are strains of *M. africanum*. This invalidates the use of this test alone for identifying *M. bovis*, but it can be used to screen for the classical human type of *M. tuberculosis*, which is by far the most frequently isolated member of the complex from human specimens.

Nitratase test

Three methods giving consistently reliable results are described.

(1) Inoculate 2 ml volumes of Middlebrook 7H9 broth (p. 59) and incubate at 37 °C until heavy growth is evident, usually for about 18 days. Add 0.05 ml of a

4% w/v aqueous solution of potassium nitrate (KNO$_3$), sterilized by autoclaving, and incubate for 4 hours at 37 °C. Add in sequence 0.05 ml, or two drops, of N hydrochloric acid, 0.2% w/v aqueous sulphanilic acid and 0.1% w/v aqueous N-1-naphthyl-diethylene-diamine dihydrochloride. (Store the latter two reagents in the dark at +4 °C for no longer than one month.) A pink colour indicates nitratase activity, i.e. that nitrate has been reduced to nitrite. Some strains also reduce nitrite; therefore, if no colour is observed, add a very small amount of zinc dust. This reduces nitrate to nitrite so that, if the strain is nitratase negative, a pink colour will appear. An absence of colour development confirms that all nitrate has been reduced and that the strain is therefore nitratase positive. Note: 'false positive' nitratase reactions may occur if the culture is contaminated by certain other bacteria.

(2) Grow the organisms on a LJ slope (not containing pyruvate), transfer a few colonies to a 0.1% w/v solution of sodium nitrate, incubate at 37 °C for 4 hours and then proceed as above.

(3) The use of a powder, Lampe reagent, makes the test easier to perform while giving similar results. Prepare the reagent by mixing, with vigorous shaking, one part of N-1-naphthyl-diethylene-diamine dihydrochloride, one part of sulphanilic acid and 10 parts of L(+) tartaric acid in a dark bottle. The mixture may be stored in the dark for up to 6 months. Transfer a loopful of a recently grown culture on egg media to a tube containing an aqueous 0.01 M (0.085%) solution of sodium nitrate and incubate for 3 hours at 37 °C. Add a small quantity of Lampe reagent (such as a knife point: the quantity is not critical). Read and interpret as in (1) above.

Controls: Positive—*M. tuberculosis* (slow grower), *M. fortuitum* (rapid grower)
Negative—*M. bovis* (slow grower), *M. chelonae* (rapid grower)

Oxygen preference

The method of Marks (1972) is used with semisolid Middlebrook 7H9 or Kirchner medium (i.e. containing 0.1% pure agar) tubed in 10 ml amounts. Inoculate by introducing 0.2 ml of the suspension about 1 cm below the surface and then mix carefully to avoid air bubbles and aeration. Incubate at 37 °C undisturbed for 18 days.

Aerobic growth occurs at or near the surface of the medium, sometimes extending as much as 10 mm below it. Microaerophilic growth occurs as a band, 10–20 mm below the surface, sometimes extending upwards.

Controls: Aerobic—*M. tuberculosis*
Microaerophilic—*M. bovis*

Pyrazinamide susceptibility and pyrazinamidase activity

It is well known that *M. bovis* is resistant to this drug. The non-radiometric and radiometric methods for determining susceptibility to this agent are described on p. 107 and p. 109, respectively.

In strains susceptible to this agent, pyrazinamide is converted to pyrazinoic acid by the enzyme pyrazinamidase. Thus, detection of this enzyme activity is an alternative to susceptibility testing for purposes of identification. Bönicke (1962) included pyrazinamidase in a set of 10 amidase assays for taxonomic studies and identification but these are rarely used now and the technically simpler method of Wayne (1979) is recommended.

Middlebrook 7H9 broth (see above)	1000 ml
Pyrazinamide	100 mg
Sodium pyruvate	2 g
Agar	15 g

Dissolve by steaming. Dispense in 5 ml amounts in screw-cap bottles and sterilize by autoclaving at 115 °C for 15 minutes. Allow to cool in the upright position so that butts rather than slopes are formed. Inoculate the medium heavily, so that the inoculum is visible to the naked eye. Incubate at 37 °C for 7 days. Then add 1 ml of a freshly prepared solution of ferrous ammonium sulphate, 1% w/v in distilled water. Refrigerate at 4 °C for 4 hours. A positive reaction is indicated by a pink band in the upper part of the butt of medium. Include control slopes inoculated with, respectively, *M. tuberculosis* (positive) and *M. bovis* (negative). A few strains of *M. bovis* produce a very faint pink band which is scored as negative.

Controls: Positive—*M. tuberculosis*
                    Negative—*M. bovis*

Cycloserine susceptibility

Rist *et al.* (1967) noted that BCG was more resistant than other members of the *M. tuberculosis* complex to cycloserine. The medium used is LJG containing 20 mg/l of cycloserine. Inoculated cultures are incubated for 28 days at 37 °C and the growth compared with that on LJG control tubes.

Controls: Susceptible—*M. tuberculosis*
                    Resistant—BCG

Pyruvate preference

Mycobacterium bovis usually grows better on LJP than on LJG. A tube of each medium is inoculated and growth is compared after incubation at 37 °C for 28 days.

Table 8.2 shows the reactions of the different members of the *M. tuberculosis* complex, including BCG. It should be noted, however, that identification of a strain as *M. tuberculosis*, *M. bovis* or *M. africanum* does not indicate the origin of the strain nor the ethnic group of the patient. These variants are widely distributed.

In practice, time and labour may be saved by including a tube of TCH medium in the initial screening tests (above). Any strain that grows on this medium may safely be regarded as the classical *M. tuberculosis*, which is the commonest member of the complex to be isolated from human specimens. The other tests need to be done only on strains that are inhibited by this agent.

Table 8.2 Characteristics of the species and their variants within the *M. tuberculosis* complex

Species and variant	Nitratase activity	Oxygen preference	Pyrazinamide susceptibility*	Pyrazinamidase	TCH susceptibility
M. tuberculosis:					
Classical	Positive	Aerobic	Sensitive	Positive	Resistant
Asian	Positive	Aerobic	Sensitive	Positive	Sensitive
M. africanum:					
Type I	Negative	Microaerophilic	Sensitive	Positive	Sensitive
Type II	Positive	Microaerophilic	Sensitive	Positive	Sensitive
M. bovis:					
Classical	Negative	Microaerophilic	Resistant	Negative	Sensitive
BCG†	Negative	Aerobic	Resistant	Negative	Sensitive

TCH = susceptibility to thiophen-2-carboxylic acid hydrazide
*These tests are not applicable to all strains of *M. bovis* as some fail to grow on the media used
†Strains of BCG are resistant to cycloserine

The niacin test

Test strips are commercially available (Difco) and are used according to the manufacturer's instructions. Isoniazid test strips, used for detecting isoniazid in urine, are also suitable for this purpose as isoniazid is an analogue of niacin and gives an identical colour reaction. Other techniques have been described, including that originally described by Konno (1956), but they require the use of toxic and carcinogenic chemicals and are thus best avoided.

A positive reaction is given by most strains of *M. tuberculosis* but niacin-negative strains have been reported (Tsukamura, 1974). Positive reactions are also given by some strains of *M. africanum*, *M. simiae*, *M. kansasii* and *M. avium*; and by some rapidly growing mycobacteria, notably some strains of *M. chelonae* (including a variant termed '*Mycobacterium borstelense* var. *niacino-genes*'; Bönicke and Ewoldt, 1965). Other mycobacteria, including *M. bovis*, give negative reactions, but there is always the possibility that negative results, obtained with other mycobacteria, are due to poor growth.

Species and variants of the *M. tuberculosis* complex

Mycobacterium tuberculosis

The classical and Asian variants of *M. tuberculosis* belong to the original species described by Lehmann and Neumann (1896) and redefined by Runyon *et al.* (1967) and Kubica *et al.* (1972).

On subculture, colonies on egg media at 18 days are 1–2 mm in diameter, rough, heaped and resemble breadcrumbs or cauliflowers. There is no preference for glycerol or pyruvate media.

The bacilli are $2-4 \times 0.3-0.5$ μm but occasionally shorter or longer cells are seen. In carefully prepared smears from young cultures the bacilli show a 'serpentine cord' pattern (see Figure 7.1, p. 66).

Growth is restricted to 34–38 °C. Both variants are nitratase positive, aerobic and are susceptible to pyrazinamide and cycloserine. The classical human variant is resistant to thiophen-2-carboxylic acid hydrazide (TCH) but the Asian variant is susceptible. Contrary to some opinions, we have found that this difference is independent of resistance to isoniazid (Yates *et al.*, 1984). Both variants are usually niacin positive though a few exceptions occur. Isoniazid-susceptible strains give a strongly positive catalase reaction but isoniazid-resistant strains often, but not always, give weak or negative reactions.

Mycobacterium bovis

Although differences between the 'bovine tubercle bacillus' and the 'human tubercle bacillus' were recognized at the end of the 19th century (Smith, 1898), the specific name *M. bovis* was not introduced until much later (Karlson and Lessel, 1970). Growth on pyruvate media is usually much better than that on glycerol media. On subculture, colonies on egg media at 18 days are about 1 mm in diameter, flatter and smoother than those of the human variant and older colonies may have raised central papillae (umbonate colonies).

The bacilli are generally shorter and may be plumper than those of *M. tuberculosis*. They are usually arranged in clumps but there is less tendency to produce long serpentine cords.

Growth is restricted to 34–38 °C. Strains are nitratase negative, microaerophilic, susceptible to TCH and cycloserine but resistant to pyrazinamide. They are niacin negative.

Mycobacterium africanum

This organism was first found in west Africa and named *M. africanum* by Castets *et al.* (1969) but strains with slightly different characteristics have also been found in east Africa. There are two major variants of *M. africanum* (Collins *et al.*, 1982).

The African I variant, principally of west African origin, is nitratase negative and, on subculture, colonies on egg media at 18 days resemble those of *M. bovis*, but may not show preference for pyruvate. The African II variant, of east African origin, is nitratase positive and colonies resemble those of *M. tuberculosis*. Both are microaerophilic and are susceptible to TCH, pyrazinamide and cycloserine. The niacin reaction of both is variable. Microscopically, the bacilli are similar in appearance to *M. bovis*. Growth is restricted to 34–38 °C.

Bacille Calmette-Guérin (BCG)

The cultural and morphological features of this vaccine strain are similar to those of the classical human variant of *M. tuberculosis*, even though it was derived from a strain of bovine origin (Yates *et al.*, 1978). There is no preference for pyruvate and, despite being of bovine origin, some strains only grow on glycerol-based media.

It is nitratase negative (or weakly positive), aerobic, susceptible to TCH but resistant to both pyrazinamide and cycloserine. There is often a minor resistance to isoniazid and ethambutol (resistance ratio 2) but this is of no clinical significance.

The history of BCG is rather cloudy. For a review, see Grange *et al.* (1983).

Mycobacterium microti

The 'vole or murine tubercle bacillus' of Wells (1946) was named *M. microti* (after the vole, *Microtus agrestis*) by Reed (1957). Only a few culture collection strains exist and the five that we have examined had the characteristics of the African I variant of *M. africanum* (Yates, 1984).

Other variants

Hein and Tomasovic (1981) isolated 25 strains of *M. bovis* from water buffaloes in Australia. These strains grew well on LJG medium and in the presence of 5% sodium chloride. Other strains with anomalous properties have been isolated from seals, cats and the rock hyrax or dassie.

Identification of other species of mycobacteria

Mycobacteria that are not obligate parasites may be opportunist pathogens, transient colonizers or contaminants in pathological material. It is important to identify them, especially when they are isolated on more than one occasion from the same patient. Although some mycobacterial species are rarely pathogenic, and some have never been known to cause human or animal disease, the distinction between pathogens and non-pathogens is a blurred one, especially in immunosuppressed people. Thus, while certain isolates, notably the rapidly growing chromogens, need not routinely be identified at species level, clinical features may, on occasions, indicate more thorough studies.

Terminology

The early bacteriologists recognized that the cultivable mycobacteria could be divided into two groups, the 'rapid growers' and the 'slow growers'. The former give a good growth on subculture on egg media within 5 days (primary isolation may take considerably longer). Most pathogenic mycobacteria are slow growers. With very rare exceptions, the only rapid growers that cause human disease are *M. chelonae* and *M. fortuitum*.

Many unsatisfactory collective epithets have been given to mycobacteria other than members of the *M. tuberculosis* complex and *M. leprae* (Marks, 1958; Wayne, 1964; Hauduroy, 1965; Grange and Collins, 1983). These include 'atypical', 'indeterminate', 'anonymous', MOTT (mycobacteria other than tubercle) bacilli, and NTM (non-tuberculous mycobacteria). A more precise term, which is gaining acceptance, is environmental mycobacteria (EM). The EM causing disease are often termed 'opportunist mycobacterial pathogens'. The term tuberculosis, at least in medical practice, is restricted to disease caused by members of the *M. tuberculosis* complex. Illnesses caused by opportunist mycobacterial pathogens are usually termed 'mycobacterioses'. In veterinary practice, the term 'avian tuberculosis' refers to disease in birds caused by *M. avium*.

The environmental mycobacteria were placed in four groups according to their pigmentation and growth rate (Timpe and Runyon, 1954), i.e.

Group I,   photochromogens
Group II,   scotochromogens
Group III,   non-chromogens
Group IV,   rapid growers.

As the names suggest, strains in Group I produce pigment, usually bright yellow or orange, when grown in, or after exposure to, light. Strains in Group II produce pigment when grown in either light or dark. In some cases, the colour is more intense when strains of this group are exposed to light. Strains in Group III produce no such pigment, although some strains develop a light lemon or pink colour, particularly on prolonged incubation. This pigmentation is, however, much less evident than the vivid yellow colour of strains in Groups I and II. The two rapid growers that cause disease in humans, *M. chelonae* and *M. fortuitum*, are non-chromogens but many of the other rapid growing species are either photochromogens or scotochromogens.

Conventional identification methods: cultural and biochemical tests

The tests described here are those that have been found to be reliable and reproducible. Most of them are used by members of the European Society for Mycobacteriology.

Macroscopic and microscopic examination

Note the colony appearance, consistency, rate of growth and ease with which the growth is emulsified for microscopy. Examine ZN-stained smears for size, shape, intensity of staining and distribution of bacilli (see Figures 7.1–7.4, pp. 66–7) and for the presence of non-acid-fast contaminants.

Preparation of inocula

Make suspensions as described on p. 71. Inoculate culture media with approximately 5–10 μl, using disposable plastic loops or a MicroRepette (see Figure 2.6 g, p. 21).

Growth at various temperatures

Inoculate five tubes of LJG and incubate one of each at these temperatures: 20, 25, 37, 42 and 44 °C. If growth occurs at only 30–33 °C on the primary culture, include an additional tube for incubation within this temperature range.

Incubators with cooling coils are almost essential for the lower temperatures and solid incubation blocks are better (and safer) than water-baths for incubation at 42 and 44 °C (see p. 19). For additional temperature stability, these blocks may be placed in the 37 °C incubator room.

Examine the cultures at 3, 7, 14 and 21 days, but some mycobacteria require even longer to give observable growth.

Pigment production

Inoculate two LJG tubes and place one in an internally illuminated 37 °C incubator (see p. 71) and the other in a light-proof box, also incubated at 37 °C.

Compare the growths after 18 days' incubation. As described above, production of a yellow or orange pigment indicates that the organism is a chromogen. Photochromogens produce their pigment only when exposed to light. Scotochromogens produce pigment in the dark, though exposure to light may increase the intensity of the colour. Photochromogenicity may depend on temperature: *M. szulgai*, for example, is photochromogenic at 25 °C but scotochromogenic at 37 °C.

Some mycobacteria, e.g. *M. xenopi*, a few members of the *M. avium* complex and *M. ulcerans*, may produce only a small amount of yellow pigment, unaffected by light. Although strictly speaking these are scotochromogens, they are usually classified as non-chromogens.

Controls: Photochromogen—*M. kansasii*
Scotochromogen—*M. gordonae*
Non-chromogen—*M. fortuitum*

Nitratase test

The methods are the same as those used for speciation within the *M. tuberculosis* complex as described on p. 72.

Arylsulphatase test

Dissolve 0.64 g of phenolphthalein disulphate, sodium salt, in 100 ml of distilled water and sterilize by membrane filtration. Add 20 ml to 200 ml of Middlebrook 7H9 broth containing OADC supplement. Distribute in 2 ml amounts and check for sterility by incubation. Inoculate a tube and incubate at 37 °C until a good growth is obtained (usually 3 days for rapid growers and 10–18 days for slow growers). Add a few drops of ammonia. A pink colour, whose intensity varies with different species, indicates the presence of an arylsulphatase.

Controls: Positive—*M. fortuitum, M. xenopi*
Negative—*M. phlei, M. avium*

Catalase test

Inoculate a butt of LJG medium in a bottle or tube approximately 12 mm in diameter ('bijou bottle') and incubate at 37 °C for 18 days. Add 1 ml of a mixture of equal parts of 30% hydrogen peroxide and 0.5% Tween 80 and allow the tubes to stand for a few minutes. The height of the column of bubbles is measured in millimetres. Record as follows: 0–1 mm, negative; 2–10 mm, +; 11–20 mm, ++; more than 20 mm, +++.

Controls: Positive—*M. kansasii*
               Negative—*M. xenopi*

Tween hydrolysis

The substrate is a solution of Tween 80 and neutral red in a phosphate buffer.

(1) Disodium phosphate ($Na_2HPO_4.12H_2O$)   22.88 g in 1 l distilled water
(2) Monopotassium phosphate (KH_2PO_4),   9.07 g in 1 l distilled water
    anhydrous

Mix 61.1 ml of (1) with 38.9 ml of (2), add 0.5 ml of Tween 80 and 2.0 ml of 0.1% neutral red. Tube in 3 ml amounts and autoclave.

Use a heavy inoculum, directly from a well-grown LJG culture, incubate at 37 °C and examine after 7 and 14 days. A change of colour, from straw yellow to red indicates that the Tween has been hydrolysed, releasing the dye. Some mycobacteria give negative reactions at 7 days but positive reactions at 14 days.

Controls: Positive—*M. kansasii*
               Negative—*M. avium*

Tellurite reduction

Inoculate Middlebrook 7H9 broth (2 ml) and incubate at 37 °C until there is a heavy growth (three days for rapidly growing mycobacteria, 10–14 days for others). Add four drops of sterile 0.2% potassium tellurite, return the culture to the incubator and examine daily. A heavy black deposit, appearing within 7 days, indicates tellurite reduction. Ignore grey deposits.

Controls: Positive—*M. avium*
               Negative—*M. xenopi*

Growth in N medium (Collins, 1962)

Sodium chloride (NaCl)	1.0 g
Magnesium chloride ($MgCl.7H_2O$)	0.2 g
Monopotassium phosphate (KH_2PO_4), anhydrous	0.5 g
Disodium phosphate ($Na_2HPO_4.12H_2O$)	3.0 g
Ammonium sulphate ($(NH_4)_2SO_4$)	10.0 g
Glucose	10.0 g
Distilled water, to	1.0 l

Dissolve by heat, adjust pH, if necessary, to 6.8–7.0, tube and autoclave.

The medium contains ammonium sulphate as the sole source of nitrogen. Add 5 μl of the suspension and incubate at 37 °C. Mycobacteria that do not require complex sources of nitrogen grow within 3 days.

Controls: Positive—*M. fortuitum*
　　　　　　Negative—*M. avium*

The properties of species that may be encountered in medical and veterinary material are shown in Table 8.3

Resistance to antibacterial agents

Tests for susceptibility to antibacterial agents, especially ethambutol and rifampicin, are useful aids in the identification of some mycobacteria. The techniques are described in Chapter 9. In addition, for purposes of identification, single dilutions of thiacetazone, 20 mg/l, and ciprofloxacin, 5 mg/l, in LJG medium are used. The susceptibilities of species that may be encountered in medical and veterinary material are shown in Table 8.4.

Lipid chromatography

Marks and Szulga (1965) and Jenkins (1981) showed that mycobacteria could be identified by using thin layer chromatography to determine their lipid patterns. The method is particularly useful for identifying unusual species, e.g. *M. malmoense* and *M. szulgai*, and for distinguishing between the various species of rapidly growing mycobacteria. The method described below was developed at the PHLS Mycobacterium Reference Unit, Cardiff, and is given here by permission of the former Director, Dr P. A. Jenkins.

Preparation of silica gel plates
Mix 30 g of silica gel (the exact amount may vary with different batches), and distilled water, 65 ml, in a stoppered flask to give a slurry that will spread evenly and is free from air bubbles. Coat glass plates, 20 × 10 cm, cleaned with dichromate solution then washed and dried, with the slurry to give a layer approximately 0.1 mm thick, using the Shandon Uniplan apparatus. Leave the plates until they have a matt surface and then dry them at 100 °C for 30 minutes in a hot-air oven fitted with a fan. Wash the plates with acetone, dry them at 100 °C and then activate them by heating at 120 °C for a further 30 minutes. They may be stored over silica gel for up to seven days. Alternatively, use commercially available ready prepared Whatman KG silica gel plates (Kodak) 250 μm thick.

Lipid extract
Grow cultures of organisms on LJ medium or in Kirchner medium, depending on which medium supports better growth. Include controls of known species with each batch of tests.

Scrape the organisms from the surface of LJ medium, or harvest them from Kirchner medium by centrifugation, and transfer them to a small glass bottle of known weight. Dry over phosphorous pentoxide in a vacuum desiccator at 50 cmHg and reweigh the bottles to determine the dry weight of the bacillary mass. At this stage the bacilli may be stored at 4 °C for several months.

To extract the lipids, freshly prepare a mixture of diethyl ether:ethanol:water

Table 8.3 Usual properties of some environmental mycobacteria that may be encountered in clinical material

Species	Pigment	Nitratase	Tween hydrolysis	Growth at					Sulphatase*		Catalase†	Tellurite‡	Growth on N medium
				20°C	25°C	33°C	42°C	44°C	3 day	21 day			
Slow growers:													
M. kansasii	P	+	+	−	+	+	v	−		+	+++	−	−
M. marinum	P	−	+	+	+	+	−	−		++	++	−	V
M. xenopi	N/S	−	−	−	−	+	+	+		+++	−	+	−
M. avium-intracellulare complex	N/S	−	−	V	+	+	+	V		V	−	+	−
M. malmoense	N	+	+ (late)	−	+	+	−	−		−	−	−	−
M. simiae	P	−	−	−	−	+	v	−		V	++	−	−
M. scrofulaceum	S	−	−	V	+	+	V	−		−	−	−	−
M. szulgai	S/P§	+	+	−	+	+	−	−		+++	++	−	−
M. gordonae	S	−	+	+	+	+	−	−		+	++	−	−
M. gastri	N	−	+	+	+	+	−	−		+	+	−	−
M. terrae	N	+	+	V	+	+	−	−		+	+++	−	−
M. triviale	N	−	+	V	+	+	−	−		+	+	−	−
M. nonchromogenicum	N	−	+	V	+	+	−	−		+++	+++	−	−
M. celatum	N/S	−	−	−	+	+	+	+		+	−	−	−
M. ulcerans	N/S	−	−	−	−	+	−	−	−	−	+	−	−
Rapid growers:													
M. fortuitum	N	+	−	+	+	+	v	−	+++	+++	V	+	+++
M. chelonae	N	−	−	+	+	+	−	−	+++	+++	V	+	+++
M. smegmatis	N	+	+	+	+	+	+	+	−	+	++	+	+++
M. phlei	S	+	+	+	+	+	+	+	−	+	++	+	++
M. flavescens	S	+	+	+	+	+	−	−		+	+	−	++

TZ = thiacetazone; P = photochromogen; S = scotochromogen; N = non-chromogen; S = susceptible; R = resistant; + = usually positive reaction or growth; − = usually negative reaction or no growth; V = variable reaction
*Sulphatase: +++, deep pink; ++, pink; +, pale pink
†Catalase: Amount of foam, +++, more than 20 mm; ++, 11–20 mm; +, 2–10 mm; −, less than 2 mm
‡Test not usually done on pigmented strains
§M. szulgai is photochromogenic at 37°C but scotochromogenic at 25°C

Table 8.4 Usual susceptibilities to thiacetazone, ethambutol, rifampicin and ciprofloxacin of some opportunist mycobacteria and others that may be encountered in clinical material

Species	Thiacetazone	Ethambutol	Rifampicin	Ciprofloxacin
M. kansasii	S	S	S	V
M. marinum	R	S	V	V
M. xenopi	R	R	S	S
M. avium-intracellulare complex	V	V	R	R
M. malmoense	R	S	S	S
M. simiae	R	V	R	R
M. scrofulaceum	V	V	R	R
M. szulgai	R	S	S	S
M. gordonae	R	S	S	S
M. gastri	R	IST	IST	IST
M. terrae	R	V	V	V
M. triviale	R	V	R	V
M. nonchromogenicum	R	V	V	V
M. celatum	R	S	R	S
M. ulcerans	R	S	S	S
M. fortuitum	R	R	R	S
M. chelonae	R	R	R	V
M. smegmatis	R	V	V	IST
M. phlei	R	V	V	IST
M. flavescens	R	S	R	S

S = susceptible; R = resistant; V = variable; IST = insufficient strains tested

(17:17:6 v/v) and add in the proportion 16 μl to 1 mg dry weight of mycobacteria. Stopper the tubes and leave at room temperature overnight.

Application
Apply a total volume of 10 μl of the extract to a plate in four separate 2.5 μl amounts, allowing each application to dry naturally before the next one is added. Apply the extracts 15 mm apart.

Solvents
All the following solvents give satisfactory results, although the first is more generally used:

• n-propanol:water:ammonia: 75:22:3
• n-propanol:water:n-butanol:ammonia: 57:20:20:3
• n-propanol:water:di-isopropyl ether: 45:10:45
• n-propanol:water:ammonia:di-isopropyl ether: 45:9.5:0.5:45

Use ammonia of sp.gr.0.880; add di-isopropyl ether slowly to the other fluids with continuous shaking.

Location of spots
Run the chromatograms for 10 cm, dry the plates at 100 °C for 30 minutes and then allow them to cool. Place the plates in a fume cupboard and spray them lightly with a mixture of 2 volumes of conc. sulphuric acid and 1 volume of freshly prepared 1% orcinol in distilled water. Heat the plates on a hotplate at

about 140 °C when the spots should appear. If too much spray is applied the spots will all be brownish-black in colour.

Read the chromatogram over a grid prepared by ruling 0.5 cm squares with a diamond stylus on the bottom of a glass dish. Illuminate from below so that the position and shape of the spots may be seen clearly and recorded.

Lipid patterns
Figure 8.1 shows a typical chromatogram. Contributions from the media are easily recognized and the phenol red in the Kirchner medium used for poorly growing organisms is a useful marker as the small amount in the extract gives a narrow band in the centre of unidimensional chromatograms run with the first two solvents listed above. Compare the patterns of unidentified strains with those of known species.

Additional biochemical tests

In addition to the various biochemical spot tests, a number of 'rows' have been described. These include the 'carbohydrate row' of Gordon and Smith (1953) and the 'amide row' of Bönicke (1962). Although employed in basic taxonomic studies, these methods are infrequently used in routine practice. Furthermore, with few exceptions, their use is confined to the study of rapidly growing species.

Carbohydrate row
The medium, in which the sugars are incorporated is an ammonium phosphate-based agar medium containing bromocresol purple which turns yellow when acid is produced.

Slopes of the media are lightly inoculated with bacterial growth from an LJ slope, incubated at 35 °C and inspected for colour change weekly for 4 weeks.

The usual sugars are arabinose, dulcitol, erythritol, galactose, glucose, inositol, lactose, mannitol, mannose, raffinose, rhamnose, sorbitol, trehalose and xylose (Gordon and Smith, 1953). For diagnostic purposes three of these sugars, mannitol, inositol and xylose, are particularly useful. Their reactions are shown in Table 8.5. In particular, unreactive strains are likely to be *M. chelonae* or biotype A strains of *M. fortuitum* which is more frequently incriminated as a pathogen than the other two biotypes.

Amide row
This row is based on the ability of mycobacteria to hydrolyse various amides into free organic acids and ammonia. Washed suspensions of bacteria harvested from LJ slopes are added to the amide solutions which are incubated for 20 hours, after which ammonia is detected by a the addition of Russel's reagent. The 10 amides usually employed are acetamide, allantoin, benzamide, carbamide (urea), isonicotinamide, malonamide, nicotinamide, pyrazinamide, salicylamide and succinamide. The most useful is allantoin which distinguishes *M. chelonae* from *M. fortuitum* (Table 8.5), and *M. kansasii* from *M. marinum*. Pyrazinamidase activity is used to differentiate between *M. tuberculosis* and *M. bovis* (p. 73) and urease activity distinguishes *M. scrofulaceum* from members of the *M. avium* complex. The technique is described by Bönicke (1962) and the

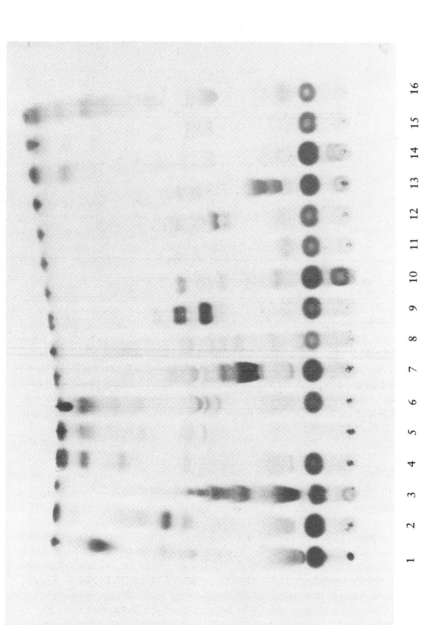

Figure 8.1 Thin layer chromatography of species and strains of mycobacteria. (1–4) variants of *M. fortuitum*, (5) *M. chelonae var abscessus*, (6) *M. chelonae var chelonae*, (7) *M. marinum*, (8) *M. kansasii*, (9) *M. gordonae*, (10) *M. szulgai*, (11) *M. terrae*, (12) *M. malmoense type II*, (13) *M. malmoense type I*, (14) *M. avium*, (15) *M. intra-cellulare*, (16) *M. xenopi* (reproduced by courtesy of Dr P.A. Jenkins)

Table 8.5 Differentiation of some rapidly growing mycobacteria by allantoinase activity and production of acid from 'sugars'

Species	Allantoinase	Acid from mannitol	Inositol	Xylose
M. chelonae	−	−	−	−
M. fortuitum type A	+	−	−	−
M. fortuitum type B	+	+	−	−
M. fortuitum type C	+	+	+	−
M. smegmatis	−	+	+	+
M. phlei	−	+	−	+
M. gilvum	−	+	+	−
M. duvalii	−	+	−	−
M. flavescens	−	V	−	−
M. vaccae	+	+	+	+

+ = positive; − = negative; V = variable reaction

simpler method of Wayne (1979), described on p. 74, is suitable for detection of pyrazinamidase and urease activity.

Additional reference techniques

There are several highly discriminative taxonomic methods which, because of their technical complexity or the cost of the equipment, are confined to a very few major centres. In general, such techniques have been used more for research purposes than for routine identification. They are divisible into three main groups: (1) the detection of antigenic differences by immunological methods; (2) the detection of structural differences by sophisticated chemical methods such as gas-liquid or high pressure liquid chromatography and pyrolysis mass spectroscopy, and (3) nucleic acid technology. The general principles of the first two methods are briefly described here and methods based on nucleic acid technology are reviewed in Chapter 10.

Immunological methods

Antigenic differences between mycobacterial strains are usually demonstrated by agglutination of whole bacilli by the appropriate antisera or by immunodiffusion analysis of the soluble antigens of disrupted bacilli. Agglutination studies are very simple and require only a small amount of culture. Unfortunately, many mycobacteria, including members of the *M. tuberculosis* complex, are rough and agglutinate spontaneously. Species in which most strains form smooth suspensions are identifiable, and some are divisible into many serotypes, by agglutination serology. In particular, *M. avium*, *M. intracellulare* and *M. scrofulaceum* have been studied by this technique (Schaefer, 1965).

Agglutination tests utilizing monoclonal antibodies bound to latex beads identify some mycobacterial species with a high degree of specificity (over 99%). Kits are commercially available for the identification of the *M. tuberculosis* complex, the *M. avium* complex and *M. kansasii* (MycoAKT, DynaGen, Inc.)

Chemical methods

In gas-liquid chromatography volatile bacterial components such as lipids are vaporized by heat and are carried by a stream of nitrogen through a column packed with a non-volatile liquid on a suitable absorbent carrier. The time taken for each component to travel through the column depends on the extent to which each enters the liquid on the packing material. Separated substances emerging from the column are quantified by ionization detectors and the height of the peaks at different times gives a characteristic profile or 'fingerprint' for the particular strain or species. The equipment is expensive but the analysis requires only a small amount of bacilli and gives rapid results. Technical details are given by Ohashi *et al.* (1977) and by Tisdall *et al.* (1979). In general, the results of gas-liquid chromatography correlate with those of biochemical tests although a few inexplicable discrepancies occur (Tisdall *et al.*, 1982).

A more discriminative, but even more expensive, technique for obtaining characteristic fingerprints is that of pyrolysis mass spectroscopy in which volatile products are liberated from mycobacteria by thermal degradation in a vacuum and separated according to their masses in an electromagnetic field. For details see Weiten *et al.* (1981). A further sophistication consists of the direct mass spectroscopic analysis of the effluents of a gas chromatograph (Yano *et al.*, 1978).

High-performance liquid chromatography (HPLC) also provides a rapid and accurate means of identifying mycobacterial species according to their patterns of mycolic acid esters (Butler *et al.*, 1991).

Species of medical and veterinary interest

The cultural and biochemical properties of species of mycobacteria, other than members of the *M. tuberculosis* complex, which are likely to be encountered in tuberculosis laboratories are summarized here in alphabetical order. Species of limited interest are listed separately, with pertinent references, but are not discussed.

Mycobacterium avium complex

This complex contains the species *M. avium*, *M. intracellulare*, *M. paratuberculosis*, *M. sylvaticum* and *M. lepraemurium*. The first two are isolated from human specimens, although *M. avium*, originally called the avian tubercle bacillus (Chester, 1901) is a pathogen of birds and some mammals including deer and pigs. *Mycobacterium intracellulare* (Runyon, 1965, 1967) is sometimes termed the 'Battey bacillus' in the older literature, after the hospital in the USA where it was first recognized as a human pathogen. In medical mycobacteriology, the term *M. avium* complex (MAC) is usually used in reference to these two species. *Mycobacterium paratuberculosis* (Johne and Frothingham, 1895) is the cause of chronic hypertrophic enteritis (Johne's disease) of cattle and other ruminants and *M. lepraemurium* (Marchoux and Sorel, 1912) is the cause of a leprosy-like skin disease of rats and cats. *Mycobacterium sylvaticum* has features in common with both *M. avium* and *M. paratuberculosis* and is isolated principally from wood pigeons.

Mycobacterium paratuberculosis and *M. sylvaticum* require media enriched with mycobactin, an iron-binding lipid found in the cell walls of most other mycobacteria, for growth. The addition of this compound to media also enhances the isolation rate of some strains of *M. avium*, especially when few bacilli are present in the inoculum.

Mycobacterium avium and *M. intracellulare* are difficult to differentiate except by techniques usually available only in reference laboratories. Thus they are often just reported as the *M. avium* complex (MAC).

On subculture, colonies of *Mycobacterium avium* and *M. intracellulare* on egg media at 14–21 days are about 1 mm in diameter, smooth, white and domed but growth may be effuse. Some strains produce a feeble yellow pigment. The bacilli are small, about 1.0×0.5 μm, often appearing almost coccoid (Figure 7.4).

All strains grow on egg media at 25 °C, most grow at 42 °C and some, particularly bird pathogenic strains, grow at 44 °C. They are nitratase negative and catalase negative or weakly positive. They reduce tellurite but do not hydrolyse Tween 80. The sulphatase reaction is variable. Resistance to all antituberculosis drugs is usual but some strains are susceptible to ethionamide and ethambutol.

They are opportunist human pathogens, associated with cervical adenitis (scrofula), especially in children, and pulmonary infections in older people. They are a common cause of AIDS-related opportunist disease, occurring in 30–50% of such patients in the USA and Europe but less often in Africa. Almost all AIDS-related cases are due to strains genetically classified as *M. avium*. Disease is often widely disseminated and, in such cases, the causative organism may be isolated from blood, bone marrow and faeces.

Mycobacterium celatum

A group of strains isolated in Finland and Somalia were found to have distinct biochemical profiles and lipid chromatography patterns (Brander *et al.*, 1992) and were subsequently named *M. celatum* (Butler *et al.*, 1993). Strains grow at 25 and 45 °C and, in common with *M. xenopi*, they are strongly arylsulphatase positive, they do not hydrolyse Tween 80 and some strains produce a light yellow pigment in the dark. They differ from *M. xenopi* in being susceptible to ethambutol and ethionamide and from *M. avium* in being susceptible to ciprofloxacin. They are usually isolated from the respiratory tract. Some other strains isolated from sputum in Finland are related to *M. celatum* on the basis of 16S rRNA sequences but show different drug susceptibility patterns; these have been named *M. branderi* (Koukila-Kähkölä *et al.*, 1995).

Mycobacterium chelonae

This, the 'turtle bacillus' of Friedmann (1903) has an interesting taxonomic history. It was at one time included with *M. fortuitum* and has been known as '*M. abscessus*' (Moore and Frerichs, 1953; Kubica *et al.*, 1972); '*M. runyonii*', (Bojalil *et al.*, 1962; Kubica *et al.*, 1972) and as '*M. borstelense*' (Bönicke, 1965; Kubica *et al.*, 1972). For details see Grange (1981).

Mycobacterium chelonae grows rapidly (two to three days) when subcultured on nutrient agar and egg medium and produces no pigment. The colonies are white, moist, soft and domed, 2–3 mm in diameter. The bacilli are about 2–3 × 0.5 μm, and some cells tend to be rather fat. They usually stain solidly although weakly acid-fast cells may be seen.

It grows well at 20 and 37 °C, although occasional strains are psychrophilic and do not grow much above 25 °C. There is no growth at 42 °C. It is nitratase negative, catalase positive and sulphatase strongly positive. It fails to hydrolyse Tween 80 in five days, but reduces tellurite rapidly. It grows well in N medium in three days and poorly on MacConkey agar, producing small yellowish colonies. Resistance to all antituberculosis drugs is usual but some strains are susceptible to gentamicin, amikacin, cotrimoxazole, erythromycin and the newer macrolides such as clarithromycin.

It is an opportunist pathogen, occurring in superficial wounds, e.g. mechanical trauma and 'injection abscesses' following the use of contaminated syringes or injectable materials. More serious iatrogenic infections occasionally occur, e.g. as a result of the insertion of contaminated porcine heart valves, following renal transplants and in peritoneal dialysis. Some cases of keratitis, usually showing poor response to antibacterial therapy and requiring corneal transplants, have been described (Khooshabeh *et al.*, 1994).

Two variants have been recognized: *M. chelonae* var. *abscessus* which usually grows well at 37 °C, fails to utilize citrate as a sole carbon source and is common in the USA and *M. chelonae* var. *chelonae* which grows less well, or not at all, at 37 °C, utilizes citrate as a sole carbon source and is common in Europe (Kubica, 1973; Collins and Yates, 1979). It has been suggested that these variants should be given the separate specific names *M. abscessus* and *M. chelonae* (Kusunoki and Ezaki, 1992).

There have recently been a number of incidents of contamination of broncho-scopes by *M. chelonae* due to failures in cleaning procedures, either as a result of faulty equipment or tap water (Gubler *et al.*, 1992; Kiely *et al.*, 1995). These strains are usually susceptible to ciprofloxacin and often only grow at 37 °C in liquid media.

Mycobacterium flavescens

This rapidly growing scotochromogen was described by Bojalil *et al.* (1962). Colonies on egg medium at three days are bright yellow, about 2 mm in diameter and may be rough or smooth. The bacilli show no distinctive morphology, are 2–3 × 0.4 μm and stain well.

It grows well at 20 and 37 °C but only occasionally at 42 °C, is nitratase, sulphatase and catalase positive and hydrolyses Tween 80. It grows in N medium and is resistant to thiacetazone (20 mg/l). Resistance to streptomycin is vari-able; most strains are susceptible to ethambutol and ethionamide but resistant to rifampicin. It is very rarely associated with human disease, but is a not infrequent contaminant of pathological material. Its natural habitat is not known but is thought to be water and soil.

Mycobacterium fortuitum

This rapidly growing non-pigmented organism (Da Costa Cruz, 1938; Runyon, 1972; Judicial Commission, ICSB, 1974) has also been known as the 'cold blooded' or frog tubercle bacillus (Küster, 1905), '*M. giae*' (Darzins, 1950), '*M.*

minetti' (Penso *et al.*, 1952), '*M. ranae'* (Bergey *et al.*, 1923; Stanford and Gunthorpe, 1969) and as '*M. peregrinum'* (Bojalil *et al.*, 1962). The species is divisible into three biotypes: A, B and C (Grange and Stanford, 1974). It has been suggested that biotypes A and B respectively should be given the separate specific names *M. fortuitum* and *M. peregrinum* (Kusunoki and Ezaki, 1992) but we are not in favour of this as it would leave strains of biotype C as an unnamed 'orphan' group (Grange, 1993).

Colonies on nutrient agar and egg media at three days are 2–3 mm in diameter, white or buff and either rough or smooth and domed. The bacilli show no distinctive morphology, being about $2-3 \times 0.5$ μm, with some fatter forms. They stain solidly.

All strains grow well at 20 °C and most grow at 25 and 37 °C. Some are psychrophilic and some grow at 42 °C. It is nitratase and catalase positive, sulphatase strongly positive, does not hydrolyse Tween 80 but reduces tellurite rapidly. There is growth in N medium and colonies on MacConkey agar are red. There is a general resistance to antituberculosis drugs but some strains are susceptible to ethionamide, gentamicin, amikacin, cotrimoxazole, fluoroquinolones, erythromycin and the newer macrolides.

It is an opportunist pathogen which may infect superficial wounds. It has been incriminated in injection abscesses, may be a secondary invader of the lungs and has caused serious problems in transplant surgery and peritoneal dialysis. It is normally resident in soil and is a frequent contaminant of cultures of pathological material.

Mycobacterium gastri

This relatively uncommon slowly growing non-chromogen was described by Wayne (1966) and is important only because it may be confused with the *M. avium* complex or be mistaken for a non-pigmented strain of *M. kansasii*. Indeed, there is strong evidence from antigenic analysis (Stanford and Grange, 1974) and ribotyping (see p. 113) that it is a non-pigmented variant of the latter. Colonies on egg media at 14 days are small, smooth, white and domed. The bacilli are morphologically undistinguished, being about 2×0.3 μm and staining evenly.

It grows at 20 and 37 °C but not at 42 °C. It is nitratase negative, catalase and sulphatase positive, hydrolyses Tween 80 but does not reduce tellurite. It is resistant to isoniazid but susceptible to most other antituberculosis drugs. Originally isolated from gastric contents, this non-chromogen is not known to cause human infections.

Mycobacterium genavense

This is an occasional cause of disseminated disease in AIDS patients (Böttger *et al.*, 1992) but differs from the more usual cause, the *M. avium* complex, in being cultivable only with great difficulty. Very feeble and limited growth occurs in the Bactec 13A medium used for the radiometric detection of mycobacterial growth. It is one of a number of species identified by unique base sequences in its ribosomal 16S RNA ('ribotyping', see p. 113). Its natural source is unknown but it has been isolated from pet birds (Hoop *et al.*, 1993) and zoo birds (Portaels *et al.*, 1996b). Other species of feebly growing mycobacteria have been identified by ribotyping and include *M. confluentis*, *M. intermedium* and *M. interjectum* (Kirschner *et al.*, 1993).

Mycobacterium gordonae

This has previously been termed the 'tap water scotochromogen' (Bojalil *et al.*, 1962; Wayne, 1970) and '*M. aquae*' (Gordon and Smith, 1955; Bönicke, 1962; Wayne, 1970), reflecting its usual source. For an account of its history see Collins *et al.* (1984).

It is a slowly growing scotochromogen. Colonies at 14 days are 1–2 mm in diameter, smooth and domed. They are yellow when first grown but on continued exposure to light the growth often assumes an orange colour. Crystals of carotene are never seen. The bacilli are 2–3 × 0.5 μm and undistinguished in their morphology and staining characteristics.

It grows at 20 and 37 °C but not at 42 °C. It is resistant to thiacetazone (20 mg/l), is nitratase negative, catalase and sulphatase positive and hydrolyses Tween 80. It is resistant to isoniazid but susceptible to most other antituberculosis drugs.

Although not normally regarded as being clinically significant it has been incriminated in human disease on rare occasions. It is found in water and is a common contaminant in cultures of pathological material; usually only one or two colonies are seen on only one of the slopes of culture media.

Mycobacterium haemophilum

Identified and named by Sompolinsky *et al.* (1978) this rare organism is noteworthy because it does not grow on the culture media normally used in tuberculosis bacteriology. It grows at 30 °C, but not at 37 °C, on LJ medium containing 2% ferric ammonium citrate, on Middlebrook 7H11 medium containing 60 mg/l of haemin and on blood agar. All the usual biochemical tests are negative. Any such acid-fast bacillus should be sent to a reference laboratory.

It has been associated with subcutaneous granulomas in immunosuppressed patients. It has also caused a few cases of cervical lymphadenopathy in otherwise healthy children.

Mycobacterium intracellulare

See *Mycobacterium avium* complex, above.

Mycobacterium kansasii

This was originally described by Hauduroy (1955) and has been known as '*M. luciflavum*' (Manten, 1957; Runyon *et al.*, 1974). It is characteristically a photochromogen, producing a bright yellow pigment when exposed to light, but occasional scotochromogenic or non-chromogenic strains are encountered. Continuous incubation in the light of the normal, photochromogenic, strains results in the formation of orange coloured crystals of carotene which are embedded in the growth.

Colonies on egg medium at 14 days are 1–2 mm in diameter and either smooth and domed or rough. When cultures are incubated on LJ medium in the dark they may resemble those of *M. tuberculosis*. The morphology is distinctive; the bacilli are long and thin, 4—5 × 0.3 μm, stain irregularly and often appear beaded or barred (Figure 7.2). *Mycobacterium kansasii* grows at 25 but not at 20 °C; occasional strains grow at 42 °C. It is susceptible to thiacetazone (20 mg/l), is nitratase and catalase positive (more than 20 mm), is sulphatase negative or weakly positive and hydrolyses Tween 80. It is resistant to strepto-mycin, isoniazid and pyrazinamide but susceptible to other antituberculosis drugs. Some strains are susceptible to cotrimoxazole, erythromycin and the newer macrolides by the disc test.

It is an opportunist pathogen, associated with pulmonary infections but is occasionally found in other sites, even in skin lesions where it may be mistaken for *M. marinum*. Its natural habitat appears to be piped water supplies and there is circumstantial evidence that infections may arise from the inhalation of aerosols generated by showers and faucets (see the review by Collins *et al.*, 1984).

Mycobacterium leprae

The cause of leprosy, this species has never convincingly been cultivated *in vitro*. It possesses specific DNA sequences and a cell wall lipid, phosphoglyco-lipid-1 (PGL-1), which may be used to identify the species. The techniques for detecting this species in clinical specimens and for conducting drug suscept-ibility tests are described in Chapter 11.

Mycobacterium malmoense

This species was described by Schröder and Juhlin (1977) and is isolated with increasing frequency in many countries. The reason for this increase is unknown but, in the past, bacteriologists may have failed to isolate or identify it because of its very slow growth and uncertain characteristics.

Colonies on egg medium take as long as 10 weeks to develop and are then very small and almost transparent. The organisms grow better after subculture and also on media containing pyruvate. The bacilli are small and have no particular morphological characteristics.

It grows poorly at 25 °C and better at 30 and 37 °C but not at 42 °C. It is nitratase and sulphatase negative, is catalase positive and it hydrolyses Tween 80, although slowly. It is usually resistant to isoniazid and susceptible to other antituberculosis drugs. It causes pulmonary disease in adults and cervical adenitis in children.

Mycobacterium marinum

First described by Aronson (1926), this species has also been known as '*M. platypoecilus*' (Baker and Hagan, 1938) and '*M. balnei*' (Linell and Norden, 1954).

On primary culture it grows only at 30–33 °C and is therefore missed in laboratories that only incubate cultures at 37 °C. It is a photochromogen and colonies at seven days are 2 mm in diameter, smooth and domed. The bacilli are 2–3 × 0.3 μm and have no distinctive characteristics.

On subculture, it grows at 20 and 37 °C but not at 42 °C. It is resistant to thiacetazone (20 mg/l), is nitratase negative, catalase and sulphatase positive, hydrolyses Tween 80 and grows poorly in N medium. It is resistant to streptomycin and isoniazid but susceptible to most other antituberculosis drugs.

It is a pathogen of fish and is found in salt and fresh water and in aquaria. It may cause superficial infections in humans, such as 'swimming pool granuloma', 'fish tank granuloma' and 'fish fancier's finger' if it enters through trivial skin abrasions. See the review by Collins *et al.* (1985).

Mycobacterium nonchromogenicum

This species (Tsukamura, 1965) is sometimes confused with the *M. avium* complex. There are very few reliable reports of human disease, but the organism is occasionally found in cultures of pathological material. Its natural habitat is not known.

Colonies on egg medium at 14–18 days are about 1.5–2 mm in diameter, smooth and domed. As the name suggests, colonies are usually white, although a pale pink pigmentation may develop. The bacilli are $2-3 \times 0.4$ μm and show no distinctive morphology. It grows at 20 °C and may grow poorly at 42 °C. It is nitratase negative, strongly catalase positive, sulphatase positive, hydrolyses Tween 80 but does not reduce tellurite.

Mycobacterium paratuberculosis

This species (M'Fadyean, 1907; Bergey *et al.*, 1923) was called Johne's bacillus after it was first isolated by Johne and Frothingham (1895). As mentioned above, it is now included in the *M. avium* complex. It can be cultured only on media containing extracts of mycobacteria (mycobactin) and isolation (from lesions in animals and animal faeces) is therefore rarely attempted.

It causes a contagious and enzootic disease of ruminants, chronic hypertrophic enteritis or Johne's disease, which is usually diagnosed clinically and by the examination of direct smears of faeces.

Mycobacterium phlei

Called the timothy grass bacillus because it was originally isolated from that plant (*Phleum pratense*), it was described by Lehmann and Neumann (1899) and by Gordon and Smith (1953). Although at one time it appeared to be common in farmyard soils and on plants, this organism is rarely encountered in the clinical laboratory. It is of historic interest.

It is a rapidly growing mycobacterium which produces a yellow or orange pigment unaffected by light. Colonies on nutrient agar or egg media at two days are 2–3 mm, rough and wrinkled or smooth. The bacilli are $2-3 \times 0.4$ μm and stain evenly. It grows at 20 °C and at 55 °C. It is nitratase and catalase positive, gives a weak positive sulphatase reaction, hydrolyses Tween 80, reduces tellurite and grows in N medium.

Mycobacterium scrofulaceum

This species (Prissick and Masson, 1956; Wayne, 1975), once termed the 'scrofula scotochromogen' is identical with '*M. marianum*' (Suzanne and Penso,

1953) but because of confusion with the distinct species *M. marinum* (Wayne, 1968) the name *M. scrofulaceum* was legalized and '*M. marianum*' disappeared into synonymity (Judicial Commission, ICSB, 1978). It superficially resembles members of the *M. avium* complex and is sometimes grouped with it to form the '*M. avium-intracellulare-scrofulaceum*' (MAIS) complex. It is differentiated from members of the *M. avium* complex by its urease activity, agglutinin serotype and by the use of nucleic acid probes.

Mycobacterium simiae

Described by Karasseva *et al.* (1965), it has also been termed '*Mycobacterium habana*' (Valdivia-Alvarez *et al.*, 1971; Meissner and Schröder, 1975). It is niacin positive and may be misidentified as *M. tuberculosis* by those who rely on that test alone and who do not incubate cultures in the light or test their ability to grow at temperatures other than 37 °C.

It is a photochromogen; colonies on egg medium at 14–18 days are 1 mm diameter or less and smooth. The bacilli are $2-3 \times 0.3$ μm and have no distinctive morphology.

It grows at 25 °C and some strains grow at 42 °C. It is resistant to thiacetazone (20 mg/l), is nitratase negative, catalase and sulphatase positive, does not hydrolyse Tween 80 nor reduce tellurite. Niacin is produced. Strains vary in their susceptibility to antituberculosis drugs.

It is associated with pulmonary disease and with disease in AIDS patients, especially in France. There is also some evidence that infection may arise from contaminated water (Wolinsky, 1979) and it may be transmitted from monkeys to humans.

Mycobacterium smegmatis

Another species of historic interest, this was described by Lehmann and Neumann (1899) and characterized by Gordon and Smith (1953). It is a rapidly growing mycobacterium. Colonies on nutrient agar and egg media at two to three days are 2–3 mm in diameter, smooth and white or buff. Growth later becomes wrinkled. The bacilli are $2-3 \times 0.4$ μm and stain evenly.

It grows at 25 °C and below and at 44 °C, is nitratase and catalase positive but sulphatase negative or weakly positive, hydrolyses Tween 80, reduces tellurite and grows in N medium. It is susceptible to most antituberculosis drugs, except rifampicin isoniazid and pyrazinamide

It is alleged that this organism was originally isolated from the smegma and generations of medical bacteriologists have been taught that it occurs in human urine and may be distinguished from the tubercle bacillus because it is acid- but not alcohol-fast. Both beliefs are unfounded. In recent environmental studies it has appeared with great rarity and is commoner in medical textbooks than in pathological material. We have encountered it less than a dozen times among some 5000 environmental mycobacteria examined in the past 10 years.

Mycobacterium szulgai

Described by Marks *et al.* (1972), this pathogen may be confused with the common tapwater scotochromogens. It is slow growing and most strains are scotochromogenic at 37 °C although a few are photochromogenic. All strains are, however, photochromogenic at 25 °C. Colonies on egg media at 12–14 days are 1–2 mm in diameter, yellow and smooth. The bacilli are 2–3 × 0.4 μm and of undistinguished morphology.

It fails to grow at 20 °C in 21 days, grows at 25 but not at 42 °C. It is resistant to thiacetazone (20 mg/l), nitratase positive, gives a weak positive catalase but a strongly positive sulphatase reaction and hydrolyses Tween 80. It is usually resistant to streptomycin, always resistant to isoniazid but susceptible to other antituberculosis drugs. It is primarily a pulmonary pathogen but infections in other sites have been recorded.

Mycobacterium terrae

This species, described by Wayne (1966), is also known as the radish bacillus as it was originally isolated from soil on that vegetable. It is uncommon but could be confused with members of the M. avium complex and M. malmoense. It grows relatively slowly. Colonies on egg media at 14 days are 1–2 mm in diameter, white and smooth. The bacilli are 2–3 × 0.4 μm, stain evenly and undistinguished morphologically.

It grows poorly at 20 °C, well at 25 °C and poorly at 42 °C. It is nitratase positive, gives a strong catalase but weak sulphatase reaction, hydrolyses Tween 80 but does not reduce tellurite. It is resistant to isoniazid. Most strains are resistant to streptomycin and rifampicin, but susceptible to other antituberculosis drugs.

It is usually of no significance when isolated from clinical material but has been known to cause superficial lesions (e.g. 'sausage finger').

Mycobacterium triviale

Described by Kubica et al. (1970), this is another species that might be confused with the M. avium complex. It grows relatively slowly on egg media. On subculture, colonies at 14 days are 1–2 mm in diameter, white and smooth. The bacilli are 2–3 × 0.3 μm and of undistinguished morphology.

It grows at 25 °C but not at 20 or 42 °C, is nitratase negative catalase positive (thermolabile), gives a weakly positive sulphatase reaction, hydrolyses Tween 80 but does not reduce tellurite. Apart from resistance to isoniazid, strains vary in their resistance to other antituberculosis drugs. It is usually of no clinical significance, but infections (e.g. septic arthritis) have been reported.

Mycobacterium ulcerans

This species was described by MacCallum et al. (1948). It grows slowly, and only at 32 °C and does not adapt to other temperatures in subcultures. Colonies at four to five weeks are about 1 mm in diameter, are colourless or faintly yellow, and smooth. The bacilli are about 2 × 0.3 μm and stain evenly. A very similar organism was isolated from an ulcer on the skin of a Japanese girl and was named M. shinshuense (Tsukamura et al., 1989). This species is closely related genetically to M. ulcerans (Portaels et al., 1996a).

The outstanding characteristic of this organism is its inactivity in all the usual tests and identification is usually based on the clinical diagnosis and the failure to grow at temperatures other than 32 °C.

Although this species was originally identified in Australia, it is the causative organism of Buruli ulcer in east Africa and certain other tropical regions. Its natural habitat is believed to be vegetation and the organism enters the human skin when it is pierced by the spines on certain plants.

Mycobacterium xenopi

This species was described by Schwabacher (1959) who isolated it from a lesion on a toad (*Xenopus laevis*) and named it '*M. xenopei*'. It was also known as '*M. littorale*' (Marks, 1964b; Runyon *et al.*, 1974) because isolation was mostly made in estuarine and coastal areas.

It grows slowly on primary cultures on egg medium. Colonies on egg media at 21 days are about 1 mm in diameter and smooth but an effuse growth is quite common. Continued incubation results in the formation of a pale, yellow pigment, which is more intense in cultures incubated at 44 °C. In these circumstances it is a scotochromogen.

The morphology is characteristic; the bacilli are long and thin, $4-6 \times 0.3$ μm often filamentous and fusiform. They stain poorly and irregularly, sometimes giving a 'lacy' appearance. Some cells or parts of cells do not retain the fuchsin (Figure 7.3).

It is a thermophile, failing to grow at 25 °C but growing well at 44 °C. It is nitratase and catalase negative, gives a strongly positive sulphatase reaction but does not hydrolyse Tween 80 or reduce tellurite. It is resistant to thiacetazone (20 mg/l) and susceptible to ciprofloxacin. It is more susceptible to isoniazid than most other environmental mycobacteria (resistance ratio of 4) and its susceptibility to other antituberculosis drugs varies. Most strains are susceptible to amikacin and erythromycin by the disc method.

It is an opportunist pathogen in human lung disease but is rarely significant when found in other sites. It is a common contaminant of pathological material, especially in south-east England, where it occurs in piped water supplies; its thermophilic nature enables it to colonize hot water systems. Human infection may possibly arise from the inhalation of aerosols of tapwater (see Collins *et al.*, 1984). It is more common in Europe than in North America.

Species of limited interest in human and veterinary medicine

This list is not exhaustive; new species are not infrequently described. Several species have been delineated on the basis of differences in the base sequence in the 16S rRNA but many other characteristics need to be described before they can really be regarded as new and distinct species. Furthermore, species thought to be non-pathogenic may, on occasions, cause disease. The species names are given here with references to their original description only.

Mycobacterium agri	Tsukamura, 1981
Mycobacterium aichiense	Tsukamura, 1981
Mycobacterium alvi	Ausina *et al.*, 1992
Mycobacterium asiaticum	Weiszfeiler *et al.*, 1971
Mycobacterium aurum	Tsukamura, 1966b

Mycobacterium austroafricanum	Tsukamura *et al.*, 1983a
Mycobacterium brumae	Luquin *et al.*, 1993
Mycobacterium chitae	Tsukamura, 1966c
Mycobacterium chubuense	Tsukamura, 1981
Mycobacterium cooki	Kazda *et al.*, 1990
Mycobacterium diernhoferi	Bönicke and Juhasz, 1964
Mycobacterium duvalii	Stanford and Gunthorpe, 1971
Mycobacterium fallax	Levy-Frebault *et al.*, 1983
Mycobacterium farcinogenes	Chamoiseau, 1979
Mycobacterium gadium	Casals and Calero, 1974
Mycobacterium gilvum	Stanford and Gunthorpe, 1971
Mycobacterium hiberniae	Kazda *et al.*, 1993
Mycobacterium komossense	Kazda and Müller, 1979
Mycobacterium madagascariense	Kazda *et al.*, 1992
Mycobacterium moriokaense	Tsukamura *et al.*, 1986
Mycobacterium neoaurum	Tsukamura, 1972
Mycobacterium novum	Tsukamura, 1967
Mycobacterium obouense	Tsukamura, 1981
Mycobacterium parafortuitum	Tsukamura, 1966a
Mycobacterium porcinum	Tsukamura *et al.*, 1983b
Mycobacterium pulveris	Tsukamura *et al.*, 1983c
Mycobacterium rhodesiae	Tsukamura *et al.*, 1971
Mycobacterium senegalense	Chamoiseau, 1979
Mycobacterium shimoidei	Tsukamura, 1982
Mycobacterium sphagni	Kazda, 1980
Mycobacterium thermoresistibile	Tsukamura, 1966b
Mycobacterium tokaiense	Tsukamura, 1981
Mycobacterium vaccae	Bönicke and Juhasz, 1964

9

Drug susceptibility tests

Chemotherapy of tuberculosis

Modern short course antituberculosis therapy (World Health Organization, 1993b) consists of an initial 2-month intensive phase of rifampicin, isoniazid and pyrazinamide. A fourth drug, usually ethambutol or streptomycin, is added if resistance to one of the former drugs is common in a given region or if intermittent (twice or thrice weekly) therapy is indicated. This phase is followed by a 4-month continuation phase of rifampicin and isoniazid. If the patient's tubercle bacillus is susceptible to the drugs and all doses are taken, cure rates of 95–98% are achievable and the few cases of relapse are almost always due to drug susceptible bacilli. For the best results, the World Health Organization (1995) recommends the use of directly observed therapy, short course (DOTS).

Unfortunately, owing to poor prescribing practices, inadequately formulated drugs, intermittent supplies of drugs, poor compliance and a lack of supervision of therapy, drug resistance is a serious and increasing problem in many regions. By definition 'multi-drug resistance' is resistance to rifampicin and isoniazid, with or without additional resistances. In such cases, it is necessary to treat patients with less effective, more toxic and more expensive drugs for long periods of time and under full supervision.

Chemotherapy of other mycobacterial diseases

Multi-drug therapy is now used for all mycobacterial diseases. Clear guidelines are issued by the World Health Organization (1994) on multi-drug therapy (MDT) for leprosy but there are no universally accepted regimens for other mycobacterial diseases. As a general rule, pulmonary disease in non-immuno-compromised patients caused by the *M. avium* complex, *M. xenopi* and *M. malmoense* is treated by an 18 to 24-month regimen of ethambutol with rifampicin or rifabutin plus a quinolone and/or one of the newer macrolides (e.g. clarithromycin). Disease due to *M. kansasii* often responds to the less intensive regimen of ethambutol with rifampicin for 9 to 12 months. Disseminated disease due to the *M. avium* complex in HIV-positive people is treated with a regimen of ethambutol with rifabutin plus a quinolone and/or one of the newer macrolides, with or without the addition of amikacin, and therapy is usually continued for the remainder of the patient's life. The antileprosy drug clofazimine was included in the original regimens but caused unpleasant side effects and is best avoided.

Treatment of disease caused by rapid growers is usually based on the results of drug susceptibility testing. Minor superficial lesions often respond to co-trimoxazole with erythromycin or clarithromycin. More serious infections require additional drugs such as a third generation cephalosporin, gentamicin or amikacin. Advice on therapy should be sought from the reference laboratory.

Drug resistance

Mutational resistance occurs at a low and constant rate in any population of mycobacteria. Thus, all patients with tuberculosis, leprosy or one of the other mycobacterial diseases must be treated with at least two drugs to which the bacilli are susceptible. If the patient receives only one drug that is effective, the susceptible bacilli are killed but the few resistant mutants replicate. If a second drug is then added, bacilli resistant to both drugs are selected, and so on.

Drug resistance, and multi-drug resistance, developing in this way is termed acquired, or secondary, resistance. Patients with acquired resistance can infect others, who develop initial, or primary, resistance.

The role of drug susceptibility testing

Methods for drug susceptibility testing are not designed merely to detect drug resistant mutants as, for reasons discussed above, these will almost certainly be found. Instead, susceptibility testing is designed to show that the great majority of bacilli in a culture are as susceptible to a given drug as one or more known susceptible strains. The object of susceptibility testing is therefore to determine whether an isolate is as likely to respond to standard therapy as one or more known susceptible strains and the techniques used to attain this goal are described in the following section.

Drug susceptibility testing is of undoubted value in the evaluation of therapeutic regimens and the planning of wide-scale treatment. It is also of value in the surveillance of tuberculosis in order to detect breakdowns in good prescribing and management practice with the consequent emergence of drug resistance. There has, however, been considerable debate as to whether a susceptibility test is essential for the management of individual patients. In some countries, a fear of litigation leads to a regular use of susceptibility testing and it is highly desirable in regions where drug and multi-drug resistance is common.

If susceptibility testing is undertaken, it is important that it be conducted to a high degree of accuracy. Much harm can be done by prescribing a more toxic yet less effective drug regimen on the basis of a false report of resistance or by trusting a false report of susceptibility rather than the patient's failure to respond to a regimen.

Even in centres with a high degree of expertise, laboratory-related errors can be made. In one report from the USA, pulmonary multi-drug resistance was misdiagnosed in nine (13%) of 70 cases (Nitta et al., 1996). The errors were suspected on clinical grounds and the authors emphasize that treatment should not be dictated by the results of drug susceptibility tests alone, but that a careful review of clinical data and other laboratory results is essential.

Methods for susceptibility tests

The high level of accuracy referred to above can be achieved only by experienced workers who appreciate the factors that affect susceptibility test results. These include:

(1) Variations in the activity of different batches of the same drug, and how this activity is affected when the drug is incorporated into culture media, which may then be heated and stored.
(2) The range of concentrations of the drugs used and the size of inoculum.
(3) The relation between the *in vitro* and *in vivo* activity of the drug.
(4) The importance of using adequate controls.

In spite of attempts to standardize the potency of drugs there is often some variation between batches and between different manufacturers' products. It is best not to change supplier, and to do preliminary titrations on each new batch of drug and on each new working solution. Some drugs bind to egg protein and the concentrations necessary in egg-based media may be much higher than those for agar-based or liquid media. Heating culture media containing drugs may reduce the potency of the latter; and storing the medium for any length of time, even in a refrigerator, may also reduce the activity of antibacterial agents.

The amount of available drug, rather than the absolute amount, must be used to determine the range of drug concentrations used in the test. We have noted that the ranges offered by some commercial laboratories are inappropriate, even missing the minimum inhibitory concentration (MIC) altogether. If an absolute concentration method is used (see below) with incorrect concentrations the MIC level reported may be unattainable in the patient's serum.

From a purely technical standpoint adequate controls are the most important factors. They must include several known susceptible strains and sufficient numbers of test strains so that deviations from normal findings may be detected. For these reasons alone the tests are not normally done in clinical laboratories that isolate small numbers of mycobacteria, but in tuberculosis laboratories at the intermediate and central laboratory levels (ACP extents 3 and 4; ATS levels II and III. See Chapter 2).

Methods for drug susceptibility testing are divisible into the conventional methods based on bacterial growth, or inhibition of growth, in the presence of a drug and a number of more rapid methods, mostly still at the developmental stage.

The potential rapid methods include tests for the detection of mutants conferring drug resistance, particularly in the *rpoB* gene affecting rifampicin resistance (p. 114). Jacobs *et al.* (1993) have described a technique for detecting viable tubercle bacilli by adding a suspension of bacteriophages into which the firefly luciferase gene has been inserted. When such a phage infects a viable cell, the luciferase gene induces synthesis of this enzyme. Luciferin added to the medium readily enters the bacterial cell, is activated by the luciferase and the cell emits light which may be detected and measured in a photometer. Bacteria killed by the addition of a drug will not synthesize the enzyme and will therefore not emit light. In addition, a number of methods for detecting changes in viability of *M. leprae*, mostly based on the uptake of radiolabelled purines or pyrimidines into DNA or RNA, have been described (see review by Grange,

1991). These could be applied to very poorly growing mycobacteria such as *M. genevense*.

Methods in current use

There are at least five of these:

(1) The absolute concentration method, which is popular in some parts of Europe, and which lends itself to automation (Meissner, 1964). A useful variant of this is the broth microdilution plate assay method (Telles and Yates, 1994).

(2) The proportion method, also used in Europe and popular in the USA (Canetti *et al.*, 1963, 1969; Vestal, 1975).

(3) The resistance ratio method, used in the UK and those countries that are influenced by British bacteriologists (Marks, 1961; Leat and Marks, 1970; Collins *et al.*, 1995).

(4) The disc diffusion method (Collins, 1955, 1956; Wayne and Krasnow, 1966).

(5) The radiometric method, which measures the metabolic activity of mycobacteria in the presence of antituberculosis drugs (Vincke *et al.*, 1982).

The first four rely on growth on conventional media and thus have the great disadvantage that there is a long delay before results are available. In developed nations, the radiometric method is used in many centres as results are obtained more rapidly.

Among the methods based on growth on conventional media, our preference is for the resistance ratio method because it uses media in screw-capped tubes whereas Petri dishes are usually employed in the proportion method and are used by some workers for the absolute concentration method. This seems to offer an unnecessary risk of dispersing infectious aerosols (see p. 28). There is no reason, however, why these tests should not be done in tubes. In addition, we describe a broth micro-dilution plate assay method which may be used for drug suscept-ibility testing and for screening potential new antimycobacterial drugs.

It is of interest that in an (unpublished) investigation carried out by members of the European Society for Mycobacteriology, there were only minor discrepan-cies between the results obtained by different workers, using the first three of the methods listed above.

All five methods may be used for direct susceptibility tests on smear positive sputum and indirect susceptibility tests on cultures. The preparation of stock solutions of antituberculosis drugs, dilutions of positive sputum homogenates and suspensions of bacilli from cultures, and the choice of control strains are the same for each method.

For a full discussion on the relative merits and usefulness of these methods in differing circumstances, see Gangadharam (1984).

Stock drug solutions
The first line drugs are conveniently prepared as 1% solutions in distilled water, except for rifampicin, which must be dissolved in formdimethylamide. These

solutions are stable for several months at 4 °C but do not thaw and refreeze the aqueous ones too often. Distribute the stocks in smaller amounts for use as required.

Smear positive sputum homogenates for direct tests
Prepare these as described on p. 61 and dilute them in sterile water. Use two dilutions, 100-fold apart, according to the number of bacilli seen per high power field in the direct smear:

Acid-fast bacilli per field in concentrate	*Dilution of concentrate to use*
< 1	undiluted and 10^{-2}
1–10	10^{-1} and 10^{-3}
> 10	10^{-2} and 10^{-4}

Bacterial suspensions for indirect tests
There are two methods:

(1) Grow the organisms in Middlebrook Tween 80 broth for 10 days when there will be about 10^8 cfu/ml. Dilute these 10^{-3} and 10^{-5} to give about 10^5 and 10^3 cfu/ml. Use the highest dilution for the absolute concentration and resistance ratio methods and both for the proportion method.
(2) Take two or three colonies, each about 1 mm diameter, or an equivalent amount of growth, from the primary culture and emulsify in 1 ml of phosphate buffer in suspension bottles (p. 71) on a magnetic stirrer. Allow to stand for 5 minutes to allow larger clumps to settle. The supernatant fluid contains about 10^5 cfu/ml and is satisfactory for the resistance ratio method.
(3) For the proportion method, make a suspension of the bacteria equivalent to McFarland tube no. 1. Dilute this to 10^{-3} and 10^{-5}.

Control strains
Include at least three freshly isolated and known drug susceptible strains in each batch of tests. The stock H37Rv strain may be used as well, but should not be used alone, especially for the resistance ratio method (Marks, 1961) as its susceptibility to some of the drugs used does not parallel that of 'wild' strains.

The absolute concentration method

This is essentially the determination of the MIC of each drug for the test organisms.

Media
The concentrations of drug in the medium must be exact, and therefore the media must not be heated after the drugs are added. This excludes egg media and the medium normally used is Middlebrook's 7H10. Solid rather than liquid media are used because cleaner end-points are thereby obtained. A very small number of resistant mutants would give only one or two colonies on agar, but cause turbidity in broth.

Use the concentrations shown in Table 9.1 and add the appropriate amount of drug to the melted medium at 50 °C before distributing it into Petri dishes or tubes for sloping.

Inoculate each concentration of each drug with 10 μl of the diluted homogenate or bacterial suspension by means of a standard loop or automatic pipette. Test each strain at least in duplicate. Four strains may be placed on one Petri dish (Felsen quadrant dishes are convenient). Allow the inoculum to dry or be absorbed by the agar by leaving the slopes or Petri dishes in a horizontal position. Tubes may then be incubated vertically. Seal Petri dishes and place them in plastic bags for incubation at 37 °C for 18–21 days.

Reading and reporting
Read MICs as the lowest concentration that completely inhibits growth or permits only two or three colonies to grow. Do not open Petri dishes but examine them through their bases. Always compare the results with those obtained with known susceptible controls. Report a strain as susceptible if it does not grow at the lowest concentration of the drug shown in Table 9.1.

The broth microdilution plate assay method

This variant of the absolute concentration method may be used to determine the MIC of antibacterial agents against all mycobacteria including *M. tuberculosis*. It is also a useful method for screening new agents.

Pipette 100 μl of Middlebrook 7H9 liquid medium containing OADC (p. 59) into each well of a 94 U-well microtitre plate. Select the range of drug concentrations to be tested and place 100 μl of a solution of the drug at double the first required concentration in the top well of each row. Double dilute the drug through the row, leaving the last well drug-free to act as a control. Inoculate each well with 5 μl of a 10-fold dilution of the bacterial suspension (p. 71). Cover the plate with a plate sealer and incubate at 37 °C for 7–10 days. Examine the wells for bacterial growth (turbidity) and record the highest dilution of drug that inhibits visible growth. The MIC is determined and reported as for the absolute concentration method above.

The proportion method

In principle, the number of colonies growing on drug-free medium is compared with the number on drug-containing medium and the proportion of resistant organisms is calculated.

Table 9.1 Final concentrations of drugs (mg/litre) in 7H10 agar for the absolute concentration and proportion methods of drug susceptibility testing

	Absolute concentration method				Proportion method		
Isoniazid	0.2	0.4	0.8	1.6	0.2	1.0	5.0
Rifampicin	1.0	2.0	4.0	8.0	1.0	5.0	10.0
Ethambutol	2.5	5.0	10.0	20.0	2.5	7.5	15.0
Streptomycin	2.0	4.0	8.0	16.0	2.0	5.0	10.0

Media
Use Middlebrook 7H10 agar containing the concentrations of drugs shown in Table 9.1. Pour it into Petri dishes or tubes. Felsen (quadrant) plates may be used: one quadrant contains drug-free medium; the other three each contain a different drug-containing medium.

Inoculation and incubation
Inoculate each drug-containing quadrant or tube with three discrete drops or 0.15 ml of a 10^{-3} diluted homogenate or suspension. Inoculate the drug-free quadrant or tube with three discrete drops or 0.15 ml of a 10^{-5} dilution of the suspension. Keep the cultures level until the inoculum has dried or been absorbed and then incubate at 37 °C, with Petri dish cultures sealed and in plastic bags, for 18–21 days.

Reading and reporting
Examine the cultures under strong light, with a low-power lens if necessary, and count the colonies on each quadrant or in each tube. Examine Petri dish cultures by viewing through their bases. The criterion for resistance is that the number of colonies on the drug-containing medium is 1% or more of the number developing on the drug-free medium. In practice, with the concentrations given in Table 9.1, there will be either no growth (susceptible) or growth on the drug-containing medium equal to, or greater than, that on the drug-free medium (resistant).

The resistance ratio method

In this method the MIC of a test strain is compared with the modal average results of several control strains using the same batch of medium. Within reason, therefore, the exact amount of drug in the medium is not important and egg medium, inspissated after the addition of the drugs, may be used.

Media
Prepare Löwenstein-Jensen (LJG) medium as described in Chapter 7 and add the drugs in the concentrations shown in Table 9.2. Each laboratory should experiment with concentrations around these levels and select six doubling concentrations. The lowest two of these should give growth and the other four no growth on tests with a batch of about 12 known susceptible strains. With experience only the three highest concentrations may be used for the tests strains, but all five are necessary for the controls.

Tube the medium, including a drug-free batch, in 2.5 ml amounts in screw-capped Bijou bottles. Place each batch in an inspissator fitted with a fan and

Table 9.2 Final concentrations of drugs (mg/litre) in Löwenstein-Jensen medium for the resistance ratio method*

Isoniazid	0.007	0.015	0.03	0.06	0.125	0.25	0.5
Rifampicin	0.78	1.56	3.12	6.25	12.5	25.0	50.0
Ethambutol	0.07	0.015	0.31	0.62	1.25	2.5	5.0
Streptomycin	0.78	1.56	3.12	6.25	12.5	25.0	50.0

*For use, select six dilutions that give near confluent growth on the first two and no growth on the other four

which has already been preheated to 80–87 °C. After about 50 minutes, remove the hot tubes and allow them to cool. We have found that such media may be stored in a refrigerator for up to 28 days without deterioration, but we do not recommend keeping it any longer.

Inoculation and incubation
Inoculate one tube of drug-free medium and one set of each drug-containing medium with 5 μl of the suspension prepared as described above. If available, use automatic pipettes (MicroRepettes) with plastic disposable tips (Figure 2.6, p. 21). Use a new tip for each strain; and discard used tips into a phenolic disinfectant or sealable disposal jars. They may be autoclaved, washed and re-used, in which case use water as the discard fluid. Incubate the cultures at 37 °C for 10–21 days.

Reading and reporting
Read the control strains first. Record the growth as CG (confluent), IC (innumerable discrete colonies), + (20-100 colonies) and 0 (0-20). Table 9.3 shows how the modal MIC is calculated.

Read the test strains in the same way. Calculate the resistance ratio of each test strain to each drug by dividing the MIC of the test by the modal MIC, as shown in Table 9.4. As doubling dilutions are used the resistance ratio is 1 (or less), 2, 4 or 8. Strains giving a resistance ratio of 1 or 2 are reported as susceptible; those giving a resistance ratio of 4 as resistant; and those giving a resistance ratio of 8 as highly resistant.

'Mixed susceptible and resistant' strains are sometimes encountered, as are 'Borderline' strains. Interpret these with caution and, if possible, repeat the tests. We confirm all resistant and highly resistant findings on new patients by repeating the tests.

The disc method

This method was introduced by Collins (1955, 1956) for screening strains of tubercle bacilli that are resistant to streptomycin and isoniazid. Paper discs containing the drugs are placed on LJG slopes that have been inoculated with test and control strains of the organisms. Some discordant results are obtained

Table 9.3 Calculating the modal resistance of five control strains for the resistance ratio method

	Drug concentration (tube number)					
	1	*2*	*3*	*4*	*5*	*6*
Strain:						
A	CG	CG	0	0	0	0
B	CG	IC	0	0	0	0
C	CG	CG	+	0	0	0
D	IC	IC	0	0	0	0
E	CG	CG	+	0	0	0
Modal resistance	CG	CG	0	0	0	0

CG, confluent growth; IC = innumerable discreet colonies; + = 20-100 colonies; 0 = fewer than 20 colonies

Table 9.4 Interpretation of the resistance ratio method for drug susceptibility testing

	Drug concentration (tube number)						Resistance ratio	Interpretation
	1	2	3	4	5	6		
Modal resistance	CG	CG	0	0	0	0		
Test strain:								
1	CG	0	0	0	0	0	0.5	Susceptible
2	CG	CG	0	0	0	0	1	Susceptible
3	CG	CG	+	0	0	0	1	Susceptible
4	CG	CG	CG	0	0	0	2	Susceptible
5	CG	CG	CG	+	0	0	3	Borderline
6	CG	CG	CG	IG	0	0	4	Resistant
7	CG	CG	CG	CG	CG	0	8	Highly resistant
8	CG	CG	CG	CG	CG	CG	8+	Highly resistant
9	CG	CG	CG	+	+	+	−	Mixed susceptible and resistant

CG = confluent growth; IC = innumerable discreet colonies; + = 20-100 colonies; 0 = fewer than 20 colonies. For practical purposes CG and IC may be regarded as equal

because of diffusion, with consequent dilution, of the drugs from the discs before the organisms begin to grow. Wayne and Krasnow (1966) overcame this problem by making the drug content of the disc five times greater than that finally required in the medium. One disc is placed in each quadrant of a Felsen plate and 5 ml of 7H11 medium poured over it. The quadrants are inoculated after the medium has dried. Recommended concentrations of drugs in the discs are shown in Table 9.5. The usefulness of this method for field work was confirmed by Griffith et al. (1971). The discs may be obtained from BBL and the quadrant plates from Bioquest (Falcon).

The radiometric method

This is now a widely used method, especially in the USA. It is more costly than the methods described above but the rapidity of results justifies this extra expenditure, especially in regions where multidrug resistance is common. The method is suitable for testing for susceptibility to all antituberculosis drugs, including pyrazinamide. In the Bactec SIRE kit, steptomycin, isoniazid, rifampicin and ethambutol are supplied as lyophilized powders for addition to the 12B medium. Also, lyophilized pyrazinamide is supplied for use with Bactec PZA medium. The method is not without problems; in particular, a mixture of

Table 9.5 Disc contents and final concentrations for the disc method*

	Amount per disc (μg)	Final concentration†
Isoniazid	1 and 5	0.2 and 1.0
Rifampicin	5	1.0
Ethambutol	25 and 50	5 and 10
Streptomycin	10 and 50	2 and 10

*After Wayne and Krasnow (1966) and Kubica et al. (1975)
†mg/litre in 5 ml of medium in quadrants of Felsen plates

mycobacterial species or the presence of a contaminant, both of which may falsely indicate drug resistance, is not easily detectable.

The Bactec system may be used to determine the minimal inhibitory concentration of a drug for an organism by inoculating bottles containing a range of drug concentrations. The more usual method is to use a technique analogous to the proportion method described above. In this method, drug-containing bottles are inoculated with a suspension of the organism and a drug-free bottle is inoculated with a 1:100 dilution of the suspension. A similar rate of growth in the drug-containing and control bottle would thus indicate that 1% of the bacteria in the culture were resistant to the drug. Full details of this proportion method are given elsewhere (Heifets, 1991; Inderlied and Salfinger, 1995 and the manufacturer's manual). A brief description is given here.

Inoculation
Harvest several colonies from a solid medium into a homogenizing bottle (p. 7), mix on a vortex for 1 minute and stand for 30 minutes to allow clumps to settle. Remove the suspension and adjust to a MacFarland 0.5 standard with Bactec diluting fluid. Prepare a 1:100 dilution of the suspension in the diluting fluid. Liquid cultures may also be used to inoculate the Bactec. Mix the liquid culture well to disperse clumps, allow to stand for 30 minutes and proceed as above. A primary culture from the Bactec system showing a growth index (GI) of 800 to 900 may also be used. (See the manufacturer's manual for dilutions to be used with cultures giving a GI of 100 to 999.)

Place bottles of 12A medium in the machine and check that they give a GI reading of less than 20. Allow the atmosphere in the bottles to equilibrate to 5% carbon dioxide. Add antibacterial agents to the bottles according to the manufacturer's instructions. Inoculate the drug-containing bottles with 0.1 ml of the suspension, and the drug-free bottle with 0.1 ml of the 1:100 dilution of the suspension, using 1 ml insulin syringes. Wear rubber gloves and avoid needle-stick injuries. Inoculate a few drops of suspension on to blood agar to check for contaminants. Incubate at 37 °C in the dark.

Interpretation of results
Incubate for 4 days, or longer if the control bottle does not reach a GI of 30 or more. The difference in GI between two consecutive days (ΔGI) after the GI of the control bottle has reached 30 is calculated. If the ΔGI of the drug-containing bottle is less than that of the 1:100 control the strain is reported as 'susceptible' and if it is more it is reported as 'resistant'. The results are usually clearcut but if the ΔGI in the two bottles are similar ($\pm$ 10%) the result is reported as 'borderline' and the test is repeated.

Pyrazinamide susceptibility tests

Pyrazinamide acts upon tubercle bacilli in anoxic, inflamed lesions where the pH is low. For reliable susceptibility tests, therefore, the medium should be acidic and a pH of 5.2 will support growth of tubercle bacilli and allow the drug to act. Even so, tubercle bacilli grow poorly on egg medium at pH 5.2 and although Middlebrook media may be used instead of egg medium the results are sometimes difficult to interpret.

Marks (1964a) introduced a 'stepped pH' method. This uses three pH levels in an enriched egg medium and one pH level in a semisolid medium overlaid on egg medium. Only one concentration of pyrazinamide (66 mg/l) is used and all tubes receive the same inoculum. Growth is compared with that in control tubes containing no pyrazinamide.

We have had good and consistent results with a modification of this method (Yates, 1984) which uses LJG medium overlaid with Kirchner medium, both at pH 5.2, but with heavy and light inocula.

Medium
This is a two-phase medium, with solid and semisolid layers.

Solid phase.   Prepare Löwenstein-Jensen medium with glycerol (LJG) as described in Chapter 7 and lower the pH to 5.2 with 5N hydrochloric acid. (Use of a pH meter is essential for accuracy.) Add 9 ml of a 0.22% w/v solution of pyrazinamide, sterilized by membrane filtration, to 300 ml of LJG medium. Add 9 ml of sterile water to a further 300 ml of LJG medium for the control. Place 1 ml amounts of the media in small screw-capped bottles and inspissate (85 °C for 1 hour) in the vertical position.

Semisolid phase.   Prepare 1 litre of Kirchner medium as described in Chapter 7, add 3 g of sodium pyruvate and adjust electrometrically to pH 5.2 with N hydrochloric acid. Add 1 g of pure agar and dissolve by steaming. Divide into two 500 ml batches and add 15 ml of the pyrazinamide solution (see above) to one and 15 ml of sterile water to the other. Sterilize by autoclaving and, when cool, add 30 ml of Middlebrook OADC enrichment or horse serum (p. 59) to both.

Final medium.   Add 2 ml amounts of test and control semisolid medium to the corresponding bottles containing the solid medium. Store at 4 °C and use within four weeks of preparation.

Inoculation and incubation
Inoculate one pair of tubes (i.e. one drug-containing and one control) with 20 μl of the suspension used for the resistance ratio method. Inoculate the other pair with the same amount of a 1:10 dilution of this suspension.

Reading and reporting
Colonies of tubercle bacilli should be distributed evenly throughout the semisolid medium in one or both of the control (drug-free) tubes.

Pyrazinamide susceptible strains give growth in the drug-free control tubes only. Resistant strains give growth in all four tubes but if there is growth in the pyrazinamide tube that received the large inoculum but not in that which received the small inoculum, report the strain as susceptible.

NB. Strains of *M. tuberculosis* and *M. africanum* are almost always susceptible while *M. bovis*, BCG and all other mycobacteria found in clinical material are naturally resistant.

Radiometric methods for pyrazinamide susceptibility tests

This has posed many problems and several methods have been described and evaluated (Heifets, 1991). The method summarized here uses materials for the Bactec system supplied by the manufacturer.

Dissolve the lyophilized pyrazinamide in Bactec reconstituting fluid which contains polyoxyethylene stearate (POES) and add to the special 12B medium at pH 6.0 according to the manufacturer's instructions. Prepare inocula as for other radiometric drug susceptibility tests (p. 107) but do not make the 1:100 dilution. Inoculate the drug-containing and drug-free bottles with 0.1 ml of suspension and incubate until the growth index (GI) reaches 200. (If the GI fails to reach 200 within 14 days, repeat the test.) If the GI of the drug-containing bottle is 10% or less that of the control bottle, the strain is reported as being resistant.

10

Nucleic acid-based techniques

In recent years, there has been great interest in the use of molecular biological techniques in the tuberculosis laboratory. The principal reason is that diagnosis can, potentially, be achieved with great rapidity and a high degree of sensitivity and specificity. Indeed, it is now technically possible to determine whether a specimen contains a member of the *M. tuberculosis* complex within a few hours and to show if it is likely to be resistant to rifampicin within a day. In addition, restriction fragment length polymorphism (RFLP) and related techniques of DNA 'fingerprinting' offer very discriminatory means of subdividing members of the *M. tuberculosis* complex and other mycobacteria for epidemiological purposes. Accordingly, there are many attractive reasons for introducing these methods into the routine laboratory. While this is very understandable, the difficulties and problems associated with these new technologies must not be underestimated. Conventional methods should not be replaced by novel ones until the latter are shown to be of equal or greater sensitivity, specificity, reliability and user-friendliness. Cost-effectiveness and economic constraints also require careful consideration as these techniques are expensive.

We anticipate that currently available methods will remain the provenance of the specialized reference centres for several years to come and that techniques introduced into routine laboratory practice will principally be in the form of commercially available, robust, user-friendly kits. In addition, this is a rapidly developing field with innovations appearing in the literature at an ever increasing frequency. For this reason, we will describe the principles of the new methodologies rather than giving detailed technical information.

From the standpoint of the tuberculosis laboratory, applications of nucleic acid-based technology are divisible into four major categories

Diagnosis
Identification of isolates
Detection of drug resistance
Epidemiology and surveillance

Diagnosis

Although nucleic acid probes (see below) have been used to detect mycobacterial DNA in clinical specimens, their sensitivity is very low. Thus, nucleic acid amplification techniques, namely, the polymerase chain reaction (PCR) and its derivatives, have been extensively investigated for this purpose.

The PCR provides a means of amplifying DNA *in vitro*. In principle, millions of copies of a single fragment of DNA may be obtained within a few hours and be readily detectable by use of a suitable probe or as a dense band on an electrophoretic strip. During cell division, the double helix of DNA is enzymically separated into two single chains. Complementary chains are then synthesized by a DNA polymerase enzyme so that two identical double helices are formed. The same replication may be obtained *in vitro* by using heat to separate the two DNA chains and adding DNA polymerase together with the ribonucleotides from which the new chains will be assembled. For complementary chain synthesis to occur *in vitro*, two short lengths of DNA that will hybridize with the two separated DNA chains must be added. These are termed 'primers' and their hybridization with the separated DNA chains forms short double helices from which the complementary chain synthesis then proceeds by extension. By selecting primers specific for a given organism, amplification of DNA will only occur if that organism is present in a specimen.

The general principles of the PCR are described in detail elsewhere (Brand *et al.*, 1991). In the established methods, the specimen is first treated to release DNA from bacilli by boiling, freezing and thawing, sonication, enzymic digestion, treatment with non-ionic detergents or by extraction with a mixture of phenol and chloroform. There is disagreement as to which is the most suitable method for use with mycobacteria. Tubes containing the treated specimen, primers, ribonucleotides and a heat-stable DNA polymerase enzyme are placed in an automated machine which first raises the temperature to that at which the double helix dissociates and then cools the mixture to a temperature that permits the binding of the primers to the separated DNA chains. The temperature is then raised to the level at which synthesis of the complementary DNA proceeds, after which a further temperature increase dissociates the newly formed DNA helices, and so on. Each cycle takes only a few minutes allowing, under ideal conditions, a million-fold amplification of the required DNA within two hours. The length of the amplified DNA chain is determined by the distance between the binding sites for the two primers on the original DNA molecule. The amplified DNA may then be detected by hybridization with a specific DNA probe or as a band of distinct mobility on an electrophoretic gel, as determined by the length of the amplified DNA product. A number of colorimetric systems for the detection of PCR products have been developed and enable the tests to be read without the need to open the tube, thereby reducing the chance of cross-contamination.

Various primers have been described for detection of mycobacteria in clinical specimens. Some detect all members of the genus *Mycobacterium* while others are specific for the *M. tuberculosis* complex, just for *M. tuberculosis*, or for other species. In some cases the sensitivity of PCR is low because each bacterium contains just one copy of the specific DNA sequence to which the primer will bind. This problem has been overcome by using primers that bind to insertion sequences (p. 115) of which there are often, but not always, many copies within the genome. For a list of PCR primers, their base sequences and detection systems see Hawkey (1994) and Butcher *et al.* (1996).

It is possible to conduct several different PCR reactions simultaneously (multiplex PCR) provided that there is no mutual inhibition of the amplification reactions. Thus, tests able to detect any mycobacterium, members of the *M.*

tuberculosis complex and the species *M. tuberculosis* may be performed simultaneously in the same tube (Herrera *et al.*, 1996).

The PCR has been extensively evaluated by many workers for the diagnosis of tuberculosis and other mycobacterial disease in recent years (reviewed by Wilson *et al.*, 1993; Hawkey, 1994; Shaw, 1994; Butcher *et al.*, 1996). These studies have revealed serious and unexpected problems with sensitivity, specificity and cross-contamination. A wide diversity in the results of a blinded comparison study from seven laboratories all experienced in use of the PCR was observed (Nordhoek *et al.*, 1994). Other similar reports of difficulties (Grosset and Mouton, 1995; Doucet-Populaire *et al.*, 1996) has led to doubts being raised as to the suitability of PCR as a routine diagnostic tool for tuberculosis at the present time. It is also important to note that PCR techniques amplify DNA from dead as well as living bacteria. Thus, they fail to give a good indication of sterilization of lesions by chemotherapy. Indeed, the technique has been used to detect tubercle bacilli in ancient skeletal remains (Spigelman and Lemma, 1993). Some specimens contain inhibitors which reduce the sensitivity of the test, leading to some false negative reports. Inhibition of amplification may be detected by use of an internal control; i.e. a small amount of DNA which is amplified in the presence of the same primers as the DNA being sought but which yields a recognizably different product. A further problem with the PCR is that, for unknown reasons, some specimens give false positive results.

The sensitivity of the PCR techniques described above is about 98% for microscopically positive specimens but as low as 50–60% for microscopically negative specimens. Thus, a negative PCR result does not exclude the presence of mycobacteria in specimens in which acid fast bacilli cannot be seen.

Certain modifications of the PCR have, however, been described and these have several advantages over the original techniques. Some of these modifications are available in robust, user friendly though rather costly kit forms, such as systems for the detection of *M. tuberculosis* based on amplification of 16s ribosomal RNA (Bodmer *et al.*, 1994; Miller *et al.*, 1994). In this method, ribosomal RNA (rRNA) is reversely transcribed, by a reverse transcriptase enzyme, to DNA which is then transcribed, by RNA polymerase (a promoter of which is incorporated in the primers), to multiple copies of rRNA and so on through many cycles. This system has three advantages: firstly, it is isothermal (i.e. all stages take place at the some temperature and a thermal cycling machine is not therefore required); secondly, it is sensitive because each bacterial cell contains about 2000 copies of the target RNA and, thirdly, the amplified products are unstable, thus reducing the risk of cross-contamination. Such systems are marketed by Gen-Probe Inc. and Roche Diagnostic Systems (Vuorinen *et al.*, 1995).

There is an enormous incentive, driven by both commercial interests and patenting laws, for industrial companies to develop further modifications of the basic amplification techniques. Frequent reference to the current literature is essential. Some newer techniques, including strand displacement amplification, ligase chain reaction and Qβ replicase systems, are described by Butcher *et al.* (1996). The trend is clearly towards one-tube systems which, after addition of the specimens and incubation, require no further handling and reveal positive reactions by colour change. Provided that problems of sensitivity, specificity, stability, robustness and cost can be overcome, such systems could find widespread application in both developed and developing countries.

Identification of isolates

Nucleic acid probes

These probes are based on the ability of single strands of DNA (or RNA) to associate as a double helix provided that their base sequences are complementary. The use of this phenomenon was first exploited for purposes of identification and classification of mycobacteria in the 1970s. In these early studies, DNA representing the entire bacterial genome was bound to a membrane and the degree of binding of radiolabelled DNA from homologous and heterologous species was determined (Baess and Bentzon, 1978). The degree of binding gave an indication of genetic relatedness, which was high within species, moderate within the groups of rapidly and slowly growing mycobacteria but low between these two groups. Although used with success in several taxonomic studies, the procedure was technically too complex for use in the routine diagnostic laboratory.

With the introduction of genetic 'engineering' techniques, it became possible to clone small lengths of DNA and to obtain them in sufficient quantity for the development of reagents. By screening 'libraries' of such clones, those unique to individual species could be selected. Thus, if such a 'probe' is added to DNA from a mycobacterial species, binding will only occur if the DNA under examination and the probe are of the same species. Originally radiolabelled, probes now incorporate non-isotopic labels.

A number of DNA probes with non-isotopic detection systems are commercially available for identification of mycobacterial species commonly encountered in clinical specimens, i.e. the *M. tuberculosis* complex, the *M. avium* complex, *M. avium*, *M. intracellulare*, *M. kansasii* and *M. gordonae* (Accu-Probe; Gen-Probe Inc). It is likely that others will become available. The probes may be used to identify mycobacteria grown in conventional media and radiometric vials (Salfinger and Pfyffer, 1994). The accuracy of the currently available probes is very high but not absolute. Thus cultures of *M. avium* (Bull and Shanson, 1992), *M. celatum* and *M. terrae* have been misidentified as *M. tuberculosis*. Identification of species by probes must therefore be confirmed by the use of established cultural and biochemical tests.

'Ribotyping'

In addition to being a useful target for diagnostic tests based on nucleic acid amplification, ribosomal RNA (rRNA) provides a means of identifying species. Although the structure of rRNA is highly conserved, there are minor variations in the sequence of bases between the various mycobacterial species. In most studies the 16S rRNA has been analysed but the 23S rRNA and the spacer region between the 16S and 23S rRNA genes have also been examined, particularly for the subdivision of closely related organisms such as those within the *M. avium* complex (McFadden *et al.*, 1994). Determination of the base sequence of the 16S rRNA has been used to identify clinical isolates and to delineate some new species, such as *M. genevense*, which grow extremely poorly on conventional media (Kirschner *et al.*, 1993). The usual method is to amplify the DNA coding for the 16S rRNA by PCR and to sequence the amplified product by a technique known as primer extension sequencing on an electrophoretic gel (Rogall *et al.*, 1990). Ribotyping has confirmed that members of the *M. tuberculosis* complex (*M. tuberculosis*, *M. bovis* and *M. africanum*) are really variants of a single species. Originally it appeared that *M. marinum* and *M. ulcerans* could not be differentiated by this method but these species have subsequently been shown to differ in a single base pair of the 16S rRNA (Portaels *et al.*, 1996a).

Rapid detection of drug resistance

Development of resistance to antibacterial agents is the result of mutations in the genes affecting the targets of the drugs (see Chapter 9). If such a gene can be identified, detection of mutational changes in its base sequence could be used as an indirect indicator of drug resistance. In the case of rifampicin, 95% g resistance is caused by mutations in the *rpoB* gene which codes for a subunit of the DNA-dependent RNA polymerase enzyme. Originally, such mutations were detected by sequencing the gene after its amplification by PCR but several simpler techniques have been described for this purpose; i.e. heteroduplex formation (Williams *et al.*, 1994), single strand conformation polymorphism analysis (Telenti *et al.*, 1993) and the line probe assay (De Beenhouwer *et al.*, 1995). Similar approaches have been used to detect resistance to other anti-tuberculosis agents (briefly reviewed by De Beenhouwer *et al.*, 1995). Research is still in progress in order to develop rapid tests for drug resistance that are suitable for use in the routine tuberculosis laboratory. For a general review of this topic, see Rastogi and Falkinham (1996).

Epidemiology and surveillance

Until recently, epidemiological investigations on tuberculosis have been hampered by the lack of a reliable system for subdividing clinical isolates of members of the *M. tuberculosis* complex. Bacteriophage typing has been investigated for this purpose but the number of types delineated by this method, although correlating with major geographical variants of *M. tuberculosis*, is very low (Grange *et al.*, 1978). More recently, technically simple and highly discriminatory typing methods based on variations in the base sequence in the bacterial genome have been developed and are being used extensively to study the epidemiology of tuberculosis and other mycobacterial disease.

DNA 'fingerprinting'

More properly termed restriction fragment length polymorphism (RFLP) analysis, DNA fingerprinting is the most widely used method for subdividing mycobacteria for epidemiological purposes. It is principally used for typing members of the *M. tuberculosis* complex but has also been used to type members of the *M. avium* complex, including *M. paratuberculosis*. The method utilizes the fact that all strands of DNA, from whatever source, contain certain short sequences of bases, usually four to six in length, that are digested by enzymes termed restriction endonucleases, thereby cutting the strand into fragments of differing lengths which can be separated by their size-related motility on an electrophoretic gel.

In the original typing methods, digestion of a mycobacterial genome by endonucleases produced thousands of fragments and the resulting gels could only be read with difficulty. This problem has been overcome in two ways. The first way is to digest the DNA and separate the fragments on a gel and then to apply a labelled DNA probe that will only detect certain base sequences that occur several times in the genome, resulting in many fewer visualized lines. These repeating sequences include the so-called transposons, insertion sequences or 'jumping genes'. Between one and more than 20 copies of an insertion sequence (IS6110) are found in almost all strains within the *M. tuberculosis* complex. The position as well as the number of these insertion sequences varies enormously from strain to strain and they are relatively stable within a given strain. Occasional minor changes have, however, been observed in sequential isolates from the same patient or in a mini-epidemic, especially in strains with many copies of the insertion sequences. On the other hand, the RFLP types of BCG vaccine daughter strains, despite multiple subculture under different conditions in many laboratories worldwide, have remained remarkably stable (Fomukong *et al.*, 1992).

Other types of multicopy DNA are also used for fingerprinting, especially when there are just one or a few insertion sequences, as in most strains of *M. bovis*, or no sequences at all. These other markers, which include direct repeat (DR) sequences, spacer oligotides between the DR sequences (used in the increasingly popular spacer oligotide typing or 'spoligotyping') and polymorphic GC-rich repetitive sequences (PGRS), are described by van Soolingen *et al.* (1994).

Technical details for RFLP typing of the *M. tuberculosis* complex are given by van Embden *et al.* (1993). In principle, DNA extracted from cultures derived from clinical specimens are digested by a restriction endonuclease and separated in an electrophoretic gel. The separated DNA fragments are then transferred to a nylon membrane by Southern blotting and DNA probes, labelled with the chromogen digoxigenin, for the IS6110 sequence are applied. The mobility of the visualized bands are compared with multiple marker tracks adjacent to the specimen tracks. The RFLP profiles of strains may be compared visually or scanned optically by a computerized reading system and matched to a reference 'library' of profiles.

The above fingerprinting method can only be applied to strains containing an insertion sequence for which a DNA probe is available. The alternative method, applicable to any mycobacterial strain, is pulsed field gel electrophoresis. In this method, an endonuclease that only cuts the DNA at a very limited number of sites is used, resulting in a small number of very large fragments of DNA. Such fragments will not migrate readily in a standard electrophoretic system but, by applying the current sequentially in a number of different directions, these huge fragments are slowly shuffled through the gel and thereby separated. This method has been applied to differentiation of strains within *M. tuberculosis* (Zhang *et al.*, 1992), the *M. avium* complex (Slutsky *et al.*, 1994) and *M. chelonae* (Wallace *et al.*, 1993).

The above methods all require cultivation of the bacilli and are therefore time-consuming. Some techniques for fingerprinting PCR products have been described (Haas *et al.*, 1993) and these can be used as screening tests for possible epidemiological clusters.

DNA fingerprinting has been used to study the spread of tubercle bacilli in mini-epidemics, including those resulting from exposure of HIV-positive people to source cases in hospitals, to determine the relative importance of endogenous reactivation and exogenous reinfection in tuberculosis epidemics and as an indirect indicator of the spread of drug-resistant tubercle bacilli in a community (Godfrey-Faussett, 1994; Stoker, 1994).

Introduction of nucleic acid-based technology into the tuberculosis laboratory

As we stated at the beginning of this chapter, nucleic acid-based technology is a rapidly growing area of research and development. Laboratories are under pressure from clinicians to introduce more rapid methods, or 'fast track' programmes and scientific and technical staff are anxious to be involved in what they perceive to be the new frontier of biological science. There is therefore a great temptation to introduce new technologies into routine practice before they have been adequately evaluated in comparison with the long established ones. While the emerging tests have the obvious advantage of rapidity, this criterion should not take precedence over sensitivity, specificity and overall robustness and reliability. Also, clinical and laboratory staff should not be 'blinded by science' but should continue to interpret the results of tests in the light of full clinical investigations. In the words of Salfinger and Pfyffer (1994): '... it must be stressed that both clinician and microbiologist have to meet the results generated by these new methods with the necessary skepticism and that an optimum collaboration is critical to a positive outcome for the patient'.

11

Leprosy

Leprosy is the second most prevalent mycobacterial disease in the world. The International Federation of Anti-Leprosy Associations (1994) estimated that, in mid 1994, there was a total of 6.5 million people affected by leprosy worldwide. The causative organism, *Mycobacterium leprae*, unlike almost all other myco-bacteria that cause human disease, is not isolated or identified in the laboratory as it has never been convincingly cultured *in vitro*. The polymerase chain reaction has been applied to the detection of *M. leprae* in clinical specimens with a high degree of sensitivity and specificity and it will probably be used in routine practice with increasing frequency (Jamal *et al.*, 1994).

The nine-banded armadillo is one of the very few animals, apart from humans, in which *M. leprae* multiplies well. Although far too expensive to use for diagnostic purposes, this animal has been used to supply large numbers of bacilli for the development of skin-testing reagents and for use in various research projects.

For more routine use, a limited growth of *M. leprae* may be obtained in mouse footpads. By incorporating various antileprosy drugs in the diet of such mice, susceptibility testing may be performed. A number of *in vitro* techniques for drug susceptibility testing of *M. leprae*, mostly based on the uptake of radiolabelled substrates, have been described (see review by Grange, 1991). Radiometric techniques may also be used for this purpose (Tomioka *et al.*, 1992) although it is rarely possible to obtain the large number of bacilli (5×10^7 to 10^8) that are required for this method. In general, drug susceptibility testing of *M. leprae* lies outside the scope of all but a very few specialized reference centres. Routine bacteriological studies on leprosy are thus, of necessity, confined to a microscopical detection of acid-fast bacilli in skin, nasal mucosa and nasal discharges. As, owing to technical similarities, such investigations are well suited to the tuberculosis laboratory, they are briefly outlined here. Some laboratories also perform histological examinations of tissue biopsies in order to classify patients according to the 'spectrum' of immune responses, as described below.

Leprosy is principally a disease of skin and superficial nerves but in patients with multibacillary disease (see below) it affects the nasal passages, from which numerous bacilli are shed, and it is probably these bacilli that are the source of new infections. Leprosy occurs in several forms which have been classified according to a so-called 'spectrum' of immune responses (Ridley and Jopling, 1966). At one end of the spectrum—tuberculoid leprosy—there is a high degree of immunological activity with the formation of tuberculosis-like granulomas containing very few bacilli and the response to therapy is good. At the other extreme—lepromatous leprosy—the relevant immune reactions are suppressed, the lesions are teeming with bacilli and the response to therapy is poor. Between these two polar forms there is a wide range of intermediate forms that, for convenience, are divided into borderline tuberculoid, mid-borderline and border-line lepromatous. As one approaches the lepromatous end of the spectrum the number of bacilli seen in the lesions, and the infectivity of the patients, increase.

Leprosy is complicated by the occurrence of the two types of tissue-damaging reactions known as Jopling types I and II. The first of these—erythema nodosum leprosum (ENL)—occurs in patients at or near to the lepromatous pole of the spectrum. It is the result of dysregulated cell-mediated immune reactions with additional tissue damage as a result of the deposition of immune complexes. It often occurs shortly after the commencement of chemotherapy. The second reaction is also cell-mediated and resembles the tissue-necrotizing delayed hypersensitivity reactions seen in tuberculosis. It usually occurs in patients in the middle part of the immune spectrum and it often leads to rapid and severe nerve damage with crippling sequelae. For more information on the clinical and pathological nature of leprosy see Jopling (1984), Ridley (1988) and Grange (1996).

Technical procedures

As outlined above, there is a spectrum of leprosy ranging from the immunologi-cally active tuberculoid form with very few bacilli through various intermediate or borderline stages to the anergic lepromatous form with numerous bacilli in the skin and other tissues. It is, therefore, only possible to detect bacilli in the skin by microscopic examination in cases that are towards the lepromatous end of the spectrum. As mentioned above, bacilli are also found in the nasal mucosa and in nasal discharges in such patients. As the latter appear to be responsible for transmission of the disease, patients with solid-staining bacilli in their nasal discharge must, for practical purposes, be regarded as being infectious. In new cases it is unusual to find bacilli in the nose if they are not also seen in the skin but they may reappear in the nose before the skin in cases of relapse (Browne, 1966). The separation of patients into those who are paucibacillary (PB) and multibacillary (MB) is important from the point of view of therapy as different multidrug regimens are recommended for these two classes (WHO, 1994). For this purpose, patients with negative slit-skin smears (see below) are classified as paucibacillary (PB) while those who are positive at any site are classified as multibacillary (MB).

The skin

Patients with suspected leprosy are examined by the 'slit skin smear' technique, in which cells and tissue fluid from the dermis are obtained from small superficial cuts. The sites examined usually include both earlobes, at least two lesions and, in the case of suspected multibacillary leprosy, two areas of apparently unaffected skin.

Clean the skin site with surgical spirit or other volatile antiseptic and allow it to dry. Pinch a fold of skin between thumb and forefinger and make a small incision in the dermis with a sharp scalpel blade. The incision should be about 5 mm long and 2 mm deep. This procedure takes some practice as the cut must be deep enough to reach the dermis, where the bacilli lie, but not deep enough to draw blood as this causes acid-fast artefacts. Turn the tip of the scalpel through 90 degrees and use it to scrape a small amount of fluid and cells from the edges of the cut. Smear this fluid fairly thickly on a glass slide, allow it to dry and fix it by passing the slide through a flame.

Stain the slide for acid-fast bacilli by the Ziehl-Nielsen method or by a fluorescent technique if the appropriate microscope is available. Examine the smear with a 2 mm oil-immersion objective ($\times$ 100) and record the number of bacilli. This number is expressed as the bacillary index (BI) which has six points, each corresponding to a 10-fold increase in the number, i.e:

1+   1-10 bacilli in 100 microscopic fields.
2+   1-10 bacilli in 10 fields.
3+   1-10 bacilli in one field.
4+   10-100 bacilli in one field.
5+   100-1000 bacilli in one field.
6+   > 1000 bacilli in clumps in one field.

It is a widely accepted belief that viable leprosy bacilli stain strongly and evenly while dead bacilli stain weakly and irregularly. The percentage of bacilli of the former type in the smear gives the morphological index (MI) which is used as a clinical guide to the viability of the bacilli and of the efficacy of therapy. In lepromatous leprosy the MI should drop from between 25 and 80 to 0 within five weeks of treatment with the WHO recommended multi-drug regimen. Not all authorities accept that the correlation between bacillary viability and staining is a close one. More accurate tests of viability based on the detection of bacterial enzyme activity do not correlate with the MI (Kvach et al., 1984). Nevertheless, there is, at present, no evidence that such tests provide more useful information than the MI in routine clinical practice.

The slit skin smear examination is repeated at intervals during treatment and gives an indication of the efficacy of chemotherapy. An increase in the MI may give early warning of non-compliance or of the emergence of drug resistance.

The nose

Examine nasal discharges for acid-fast bacilli simply by staining and examining smears as though they were sputum. Examine the mucosa by scraping the nasal septum or the lower turbinate with a small curette (Downs Surgical Limited: see Jopling, 1984). Alternatively, make a simple disposable scraper by straightening a paperclip and hammering one end flat. Spread the scraping on a slide for staining.

Biopsies

When no bacilli are detectable and when the diagnosis remains in doubt a biopsy of a representative lesion is indicated; for which purpose remove an ellipse of skin, of about 12 $\times$ 3 mm and including the full thickness of the dermis, under local anaesthetic. Punch biopsies are less satisfactory. Place the biopsy in a fixative, preferably one containing mercuric chloride, such as Ridley's solution

Mercuric chloride	2 g
Formalin (40% formaldehyde)	10 ml
Glacial acetic acid	30 ml
Water	to 100 ml

Dissolve the mercuric chloride in water by heat, allow to cool and add the other ingredients.

Leave the biopsy in this for 24 hours and then transfer to 70% alcohol without rinsing. Prepare sections for staining by the ZN method.

The examination of skin biopsies requires considerable experience, judgment and skill and lies outside the scope of this book. For full details see Ridley (1988).

References

Advisory Committee on Dangerous Pathogens (1995) *Categorization of biological agents according to hazard and categories of containment*, 4th edn. Health and Safety Commission. Sudbury: HSE Books

Allen, B.W. (1981) Survival of tubercle bacilli in heat-fixed sputum smears. *Journal of Clinical Pathology*, **34**, 719–722

Allen, B.W. and Darell, J.H. (1983) Contamination of specimen container surfaces during sputum collection. *Journal of Clinical Pathology*, **36**, 479–481

Allen, B.W. and Hinkes, W.F. (1982) Koch's stain for tubercle bacilli. *Bulletin of the International Union Against Tuberculosis*, **57**, 190–192

Allen, B.W., Mitchison, D.A., Darbyshire, J., *et al.* (1983) Examination of operation specimens from patients with spinal tuberculosis for tubercle bacilli. *Journal of Clinical Pathology*, **36**, 662–666

American Thoracic Society (1983) Levels of laboratory services for mycobacterial disease. *American Review of Respiratory Disease*, **128**, 213

Aronson, J.D. (1926) Spontaneous tuberculosis in salt water fish. *Journal of Infectious Diseases*, **39**, 315–320

Ausina, V., Luquin, M.F., Garciá-Barceló, M. *et al.* (1992) *Mycobacterium alvi* sp. nov. *International Journal of Systematic Bacteriology*, **42**, 529–535

Azadian, B.S., Beck, A., Curtis, J.R. *et al.* (1981) Disseminated infection with *Mycobacterium chelonei* in a haemodialysis patient. *Tubercle*, **62**, 281–284

Baess, I. and Bentzon, M.W. (1978) Deoxyribonucleic acid hybridization between different species of mycobacteria. *Acta Pathologica et Microbiologica Scandinavica*; **86B**, 71–76

Baker, J.A. and Hagan, W.A. (1938) Tuberculosis of the Mexican flatfish (*Platypoecilus maculatus*). *Journal of Infectious Diseases*, **70**, 248–252

Bergey, D.H., Harrison, F.C., Breed, R.S. *et al.* (1923) *Manual of Determinative Bacteriology*, 1st edn. Baltimore: Williams & Wilkins

Bishop, P.J. and Neumann, G. (1970) The history of the Ziehl-Nielsen stain. *Tubercle*, **51**, 196–206

Bodmer, T., Gurtner, A., Schöpfer, K. and Matter, L. (1994) Screening of respiratory tract specimens for the presence of *Mycobacterium tuberculosis* by use of the Gen-Probe Amplified Mycobacterium Direct Test. *Journal of Clinical Microbiology* **32**, 1483–1487

Bojalil, L.F., Cerbon, J. and Trujillo, J. (1962) Adansonian classification of mycobacteria. *Journal of General Microbiology*, **28**, 333–346

Bönicke, R. (1962) Report on identification of mycobacteria by biochemical methods. *Bulletin of the International Union Against Tuberculosis*, **32**, 13–68

Bönicke, R. (1965) Beschreibung der neuen Species *Mycobacterium borstelense* n.sp. *Zentralblatt für Bakteriologie, Parasitenkunde, Infektionskrankheiten und Hygiene*, Abteilung I Originale, **196**, 535–538

Bönicke, R. and Ewoldt, A. (1965) Quantitative Untersuchung über das Niacinbildungvermogen von *Mycobacterium borstelense* var. *niacinogenes*. *Beitrage zur Klinik der Tuberkulose*, **130**, 149–154

Bönicke, R. and Juhasz, E. (1964) Beschreibung der neuen Species *Mycobacterium vaccae* n.sp.

Zentralblatt für Bakteriologie, Parasitenkunde, Infektionskrankheiten und Hygiene, Abteilung I Originale, **192**, 133–135

Böttger, E.C., Teske, A., Kirschner, P., *et al.* (1992) Disseminated '*Mycobacterium genavense*' infection in patients with AIDS. *Lancet* **340**: 76–80

Brand, N.J., Vallins, W.J., Yacoub, M. and Barton, P.J.R. (1991) The polymerase chain reaction and its application to basic research in molecular biology. In *Genetic manipulation: techniques and applications*. Grange JM, Fox A, Morgan NL. (eds). Oxford: Blackwell. pp. 279–293

Brander, E., Jantzen, E., Huttunen, R., *et al.* (1992) Characterization of a distinct group of slowly growing mycobacteria by biochemical tests and lipid analysis. *Journal of Clinical Microbiology* **30**, 1972–1975

British Standards Institution (1988) *BS 6642: Specification for Disposable Refuse Sacks made of Polythene*. London: BSI

British Standards Institution (1990) *BS 7320: Specification for Sharps Containers*. London: BSI

Browne, S.G. (1966) The value of nasal smears in lepromatous leprosy. *International Journal of Leprosy*, **34**, 23–26

Bull, T.J. and Shanson, D.C. (1992) Rapid misdiagnosis by *Mycobacterium avium-intracellulare* masquerading as tuberculosis in PCR/DNA probe tests. *Lancet* **340**, 1360

Butcher, P.D., Hutchinson, N.A., Doran, T.J. and Dale, J.W. (1996) The application of molecular techniques to the diagnosis and epidemiology of mycobacterial diseases. *Journal of Applied Bacteriology*, **81**, 53S–71S

Butler, W.R., Jost, K.C. and Kilburn, J.O. (1991) Identification of mycobacteria by high-performance liquid chromatography. *Journal of Clinical Microbiology*, **29**, 2468–2472

Butler, W.R., O'Connor, S.P., Yakrus, M.A., *et al.* (1993) *Mycobacterium celatum* sp. nov. *International Journal of Systematic Bacteriology* **43**, 1540–1550

Canetti, G., Rist, N. and Grosset, J. (1963) Mesure de la sensibilite du bacille tuberculeux aux drogues antibacillaires par la methode des proportions: methodologie, criteries de rèsistance, resultats, interpretations. *Revue de la tuberculose et de Pneumonologie*, **27**, 217–272

Canetti, G., Fox, W., Khomenko, A. *et al.* (1969) Advances in techniques of testing mycobacterial drug sensitivity and the use of sensitivity tests in tuberculosis control programmes. *Bulletin of the World Health Organization*, **41**, 21–43

Casals, M. and Calero, J.R. (1974) *Mycobacterium gadium* sp. nov. A new species of rapidly growing mycobacteria. *Tubercle*, **55**, 299–308

Castets, M., Rist, N. and Boisvert, H. (1969) La variété africaine du bacille tuberculeux humain. *Medicine d'Afrique Noir*, **16**, 321–322

Chamoiseau, G. (1979) Etiology of farcy in African bovines: nomenclature of the causal organisms *Mycobacterium farcinogenes* Chamoiseau and *Mycobacterium senegalense* (Chamoiseau) comb. nov. *International Journal of Systemic Bacteriology*, **29**, 407–410

Cheesbrough, M. (1984) *Medical Laboratory Manual for Tropical Countries*, Vol 2. Doddington: Tropical Health Technology

Cheney, J.E. and Collins, C.H. (1995) Formaldehyde disinfection in laboratories: limitations and hazards. *British Journal of Biomedical Science*, **52**, 195–201

Chester, F.D. (1901) *A Manual of Determinative Bacteriology*. New York: MacMillan. p. 356

Chretien, J. (1990) Tuberculosis and HIV. The cursed duet. *Bulletin of the International Union Against Tuberculosis and Lung Disease* **65(1)**, 25–28

Clancy, J.K., Allen, B.W., Rogers, D.T. *et al.* (1976) Comparison of machine and manual staining of direct smears for acid-fast bacilli by fluorescence microscopy. *Journal of Clinical Pathology*, **29**, 931–933

Cohn, M.L., Waggoner, R.F. and McClatchy, J.K. (1968) The 7H11 medium for the culture of mycobacteria. *American Review of Respiratory Disease*, **98**, 295–296

Collins, C.H. (1951) The effect of mechanical shaking on the concentration of sputum for the cultivation of tubercle bacilli. *Journal of Medical Laboratory Technology*, **9**, 217–219

Collins, C.H. (1955) A streptomycin disc technique for screening resistant strains of tubercle bacilli. *Tubercle*, **36**, 182–187

Collins, C.H. (1956) A disc screening technique for isoniazid-resistant strains of tubercle bacilli. *Tubercle*, **37**, 23–25

Collins, C.H. (1962) The classification of 'anonymous' acid-fast bacilli from human source. *Tubercle*, **43**, 292–298

Collins, C.H. (1993) *Laboratory-Acquired Infections*. 3rd edn. Oxford: Butterworth–Heinemann

Collins, C.H. (1994) Opinion: Infected laboratory waste. *Letters in Microbiology*, **19**, 61–62

Collins, C.H. and Yates, M.D. (1979) Hydroxylamine and salt tolerance in screening and identifying mycobacteria. *Tubercle*, **60**, 91–94

Collins, C.H., Yates, M.D. and Down, G.F. (1981) False positive direct films in tuberculosis bacteriology. *Medical Laboratory Science*, **38**, 129–131

Collins, C.H., Yates, M.D. and Grange, J.M. (1982) Subdivision of *Mycobacterium tuberculosis* into five variants for epidemiological purposes: methods and nomenclature. *Journal of Hygiene*, **89**, 235–242

Collins, C.H., Grange, J.M. and Yates, M.D. (1984) A review: mycobacteria in water. *Journal of Applied Bacteriology*, **57**, 193–211

Collins, C.H., Grange, J.M., Noble, W.C. and Yates, M.D. (1985) *Mycobacterium marinum* infections in man. *Journal of Hygiene*, **94**, 135–149

Collins, C.H., Lyne, P.M. and Grange, J.M. (1995) *Collins and Lyne's Microbiological Methods*. 7th edn. Oxford: Butterworth–Heinemann

Commission of the European Communities (1990) Council Directive on the protection of workers from the risks related to exposure to biological agents at work. *Official Journal of the European Communities L374 of 31 December 1990*

Da Costa Cruz, J.C. (1938) *Mycobacterium fortuitum*: un novo bacilo acidoresistante patogenico pava a homen. *Acta Medico Rio de Janeiro*, **1**, 289–301

Darzins, E. (1950) Tuberculose das gias (*Leptodactylus pentadactylus*). *Archivos do Instituto Brasileiro para investigaçã o da Tuberculose*, **9**, 29–37

De Beenhouwer, H., Lhiang, Z., Jannes, G. *et al.* (1995) Rapid detection of rifampicin resistance in sputum and biopsy specimens from tuberculosis patients by PCR and line probe assay. *Tubercle and Lung Disease* **76**, 425–430

Department of Health and Social Security (1970) *Precautions against Tuberculosis Infection in the Diagnostic Laboratory*. London: HMSO

Department of Health and Social Security (1978) *A Code of Practice for the Prevention of Infection in Clinical Laboratories and Post Mortem Rooms*. London: HMSO

Dominguez, J.M. and Vivas, R.S. (1977) Smear-positive and culture-negative results in routine sputum investigations for the detection and therapy control of tuberculosis. *Tubercle*, **58**, 217–220

Doucet-Populaire, F., Lalande, V., Carpentier, E. *et al.* (Azay Mycobacteria Study Group) (1996) A blind study of the polymerase chain reaction for the detection of *Mycobacterium tuberculosis* DNA. *Tubercle and Lung Disease*, **77**, 358–362

Eidus, L., Diena, B.B. and Greenberg, L. (1960) The use of *p*-nitro acetylamino-propiophenone (NAP) in the differentiation of mycobacteria. *American Review of Respiratory Disease*, **81**, 759–760

Engbaek, H.C., Vergmann, B. and Bunch-Christensen, K. (1977) Pulmonary tuberculosis due to BCG in a technician employed in a BCG laboratory. *Bulletin of the World Health Organization*, **55**, 517–520

Fodor, T. (1984) Bulk staining of sputum by the Ziehl-Nielsen method. *Tubercle*, **65**, 123–125

Fodor, T. (1995) Detection of mycobacteria in sputum smears prepared by cytocentrifugation. *Tubercle and Lung Disease*, **76**, 273–274

Fomukong, N.G., Dale, J.W., Osborn, T.W. and Grange, J.M. (1992) Use of gene probes based on the insertion sequence IS986 to differentiate between BCG vaccine strains. *Journal of Applied Bacteriology*, **72**, 126–133

Friedmann, F.F. (1903) Der Schildkrötentuberkelbacillus, seine Züchtung, Biologie und Pathogenität. *Zentralblatt für Bakteriologie, Parasitenkunde und Infektionskrankheiten*, Abteilung I, Originale, **34**, 647–658

Gangadharam, P.R.J. (1984) *Drug Resistance in Mycobacteria*. Boca Raton: CRC Press

George, R.H. (1988) The prevention and control of mycobacterial infections in hospitals. *Journal of Hospital Infection*, **11** (Supplement A), 386–392.

Godfrey-Faussett, P. (1994) DNA fingerprinting: a powerful new tool for the study of tuberculosis. In *Clinical Tuberculosis*. Davies PDO. (ed.) London: Chapman and Hall. pp. 391–400

Gordon, R.E. and Smith, M.M. (1953) Rapidly-growing acid-fast bacteria. 1. Species descriptions of *Mycobacterium phlei* Lehmann and Neumann and *Mycobacterium smegmatis* (Trevisan) Lehmann and Neumann. *Journal of Bacteriology*, **66**, 41–48

Gordon, R.E. and Smith, M.M. (1955) Rapidly-growing acid-fast bacteria. II. Species descriptions of *Mycobacterium fortuitum* Cruz. *Journal of Bacteriology*, **69**, 502–507

Grange, J.M. (1981) *Mycobacterium chelonei. Tubercle*, **62**, 273–276

Grange, J.M. (1991) Detection of drug resistance in *Mycobacterium leprae* and the design of treatment regimens for leprosy. In Heifets L, ed. *Drug Susceptibility in the Chemotherapy of Mycobacterial Infections*. Boca Raton: CRC Press, pp. 161–77

Grange, J.M. (1992) Mycobacterial infections following heart valve replacement. *Journal of Heart Valve Disease*, **1**, 102–109

Grange, J.M. (1993) The third biovariant of *Mycobacterium fortuitum. Tubercle and Lung Disease*, **74**, 349

Grange, J.M. (1996) *Mycobacteria and Human Disease*, 2nd edn. London: Arnold

Grange, J.M., Aber, V.R., Allen, B.W. *et al.* (1978) The correlation of bacteriophage types of *Mycobacterium tuberculosis* with guinea-pig virulence and *in vitro*-indicators of virulence. *Journal of General Microbiology*, **108**, 1–7.

Grange, J.M. and Collins, C.H. (1983) Mycobacterial pathogenicity and nomenclature: the 'nyrocine' mycobacteria. *Tubercle*, **64**, 141–142

Grange, J.M., Gibson, J., Osborn, T.W. *et al.* (1983) What is BCG? *Tubercle*, **64**, 129–139

Grange, J.M., Noble, W.C., Yates, M.D. and Collins, C.H. (1988) Inoculation mycobacterioses. *Clinical and Experimental Dermatology*, **13**, 211–220

Grange, J.M. and Stanford, J.L. (1974) A re-evaluation of *Mycobacterium fortuitum* (synonym *Mycobacterium ranae*). *International Journal of Systematic Bacteriology*, **24**, 320–329

Griffith, M., Matajack, M.L., Bissett, M.L. and Wood, R.M. (1971) Cooperative field tests of drug impregnated discs for the sensitivity testing of mycobacteria. *American Review of Respiratory Disease*, **103**, 423–426.

Grosset, J. and Mouton, Y. (1995) Is PCR a useful tool for the diagnosis of tuberculosis in 1995? *Tubercle and Lung Disease* **76**, 183–184

Gubler, J.G.H., Salfinger, M. and Von Graevenitz A. (1992) Pseudoepidemic of non-tuberculous mycobacteria due to a contaminated bronchoscope cleaning machine – report of an outbreak and a review of the literature. *Chest*, **101**, 1245–1249

Haas, W.H., Butler, W.R., Woodley, C.L. and Crawford, J.T. (1993) Mixed-linker polymerase chain reaction: a new method for rapid fingerprinting of isolates of the *Mycobacterium tuberculosis* complex. *Journal of Clinical Microbiology* **31**, 1293–1298

Harrington, R. and Karlson, A.G. (1966) Differentiation between *Mycobacterium tuberculosis* and *M. bovis* by *in vitro* procedures. *American Journal of Veterinary Research*, **27**, 1193–1196

Harrington, J.A., Gill, F.S., Aw, T.C. *et al.* (1992) *Pocket Consultant in Occupational Health*, 3rd edn. Oxford: Blackwell Scientific Publications

Hauduroy, P. (1955) *Derniers Aspects du Monde des Mycobacteries*. Paris: Masson

Hauduroy, P. (1965) Terminology for yet-unclassified mycobacteria. *American Review of Respiratory Disease*, **91**, 774

Hawkey, P.M. (1994) The role of polymerase chain reaction in the diagnosis of mycobacterial infections. *Revues of Medical Microbiology*, **5**, 21–32

Heifets, L.B. (1991) Drug susceptibility tests in the management of chemotherapy of tuberculosis. In *Drug susceptibility in the chemotherapy of mycobacterial infections*. (Heifets, L.B., Ed). Boca Raton, CRC Press. pp 89–121

Hein, W.R. and Tomasovic, A.A. (1981) An abattoir survey of tuberculosis in feral buffaloes. *Australian Veterinary Journal*, **57**, 543–547

Herrera, E.A., Pérez, O. and Segovia, M. (1996) Differentiation between *Mycobacterium tuberculosis* and *Mycobacterium bovis* by a multiplex-polymerase chain reaction. *Journal of Applied Bacteriology*, **80**, 596–604

Hollerström, V.E. and Hard, S. (1953) A fatality from BCG vaccination. *Acta Dermatologica et Veneriologica Scandinavica*, **33**, 159–160

Hoop, R.K., Böttger, E.C., Ossent, P. and Salfinger, M. (1993) Mycobacteriosis due to *Mycobacterium genavense* in six pet birds. *Journal of Clinical Microbiology* **31**: 990–993

Inderlied, C.B. and Salfinger, M. (1995) Antimicrobial agents and susceptibility tests: mycobacteria. In *Manual of Clinical Microbiology*, 6th edn. (Murray P.R., ed.) Washington DC: ASM Press. pp. 1385–1404

International Federation of Anti-leprosy Associations (1994) Elimination of leprosy. *Leprosy Review*, **65**, 165–166

Jacobs, W.R., Barletta, R.G, Udani, R. *et al.* (1993) Rapid assessment of drug susceptibilites of *Mycobacterium tuberculosis* by means of luciferase reporter phages. *Science*, **260**, 819–822

Jamal, S., Wilson, S.M., Hackett, M., *et al.* (1994) A colorimetric PCR method for the detection of *M. leprae* in biopsies from leprosy patients. *International Journal of Leprosy*, **62**, 512–520

Jenkins, P.A. (1981) Lipid analysis for the identification of mycobacteria: an appraisal. *Reviews of Infectious Diseases*, **3**, 862–866

Johne, H.H. and Frothingham, L. (1895) Ein eigentumlicher Fall von Tuberculose beim Rind. *Deutsche Zeitschrift für Tiermedizin und Vergleichende Pathologie*, **21**, 438–454

Jones, B.P.C. (1995) Fumigation and management of containment level 3 facilities. *PHLS Microbiology Digest*, 12, 169–171

Jopling, W.H. (1984) *Handbook of Leprosy*. 3nd edn. London: Heinemann

Judicial Commission, International Committee on Systematic Bacteriology (1974) Opinion 51. Conservation of the epithet *fortuitum* in the combination *Mycobacterium fortuitum* Da Costa Cruz. *International Journal of Systematic Bacteriology*, **24**, 552

Judicial Commission, International Committee on Systematic Bacteriology (1978) Opinion 53. Rejection of the species name *Mycobacterium marianum* Penso 1953. *International Journal of Systematic Bacteriology*, **28**, 334

Karasseva, V., Weiszfeiler, J. and Krasnay, E. (1965) Occurrence of atypical mycobacteria in *Macacus rhesus. Acta Microbiologica Academicae Scientiarum Hungarica*, **12**, 275–282

Karlson, A.G. and Lessel, E.F. (1970) *Mycobacterium bovis* nom. nov. *International Journal of Systematic Bacteriology*, **20**, 273–282

Kazda, J. (1980) *Mycobacterium sphagni* sp. nov. *International Journal of Systematic Bacteriology*, **30**, 77–81

Kazda, J. and Müller, K. (1979) *Mycobacterium komossense* sp. nov. *International Journal of Systematic Bacteriology*, **29**, 361–365

Kazda, J., Stackebrandt, E., Smida, J. *et al.* (1990) *Mycobacterium cooki* sp. nov. *International Journal of Systematic Bacteriology*, **40**, 217–223

Kazda, J., Müller, H.-J., Stackebrandt, E. *et al.* (1992) *Mycobacterium madagascariense* sp. nov. *International Journal of Systematic Bacteriology*, **42**, 524–528

Kazda, J., Cooney, R., Monaghan, M. *et al.* (1993) *Mycobacterium hiberniae* sp. nov. *International Journal of Systematic Bacteriology*, **43**, 352–357

Khooshabeh, R., Grange J.M., Yates, M.D. *et al.* (1994) A case report of *Mycobacterium chelonae* keratitis and a review of mycobacterial infections of the eye. *Tubercle and Lung Disease*, **75**, 377–382

Kiehn, T.E. and Cammarata, R. (1988) Comparative recoveries of *Mycobacterium avium–M. intracellulare* from isolator lysis-centrifugation and BACTEC 13A blood culture systems. *Journal of Clinical Microbiology*, **26**, 760–761

Kiely, J.L., Sheehan, S., Cryan, B. and Bredin, C.P. (1995) Isolation of *Mycobacterium chelonae* in a bronchoscopy unit and its subsequent eradication. *Tubercle and Lung Disease*, **76**, 163–167

Kirschner, P., Springer, B., Vogel, U. *et al.* (1993) Genotypic identification of mycobacteria by nucleic acid sequence determination: report of a 2-year experience in a clinical laboratory. *Journal of Clinical Microbiology*, **31**, 2882–2889

Koch, R. (1882) Die Aetiologie der Tuberculose. *Berliner Klinische Wochenschrift*, **19**, 221–230

Kochi, A. (1991) The global tuberculosis situation and the new control strategy of the World Health Organisation. *Tubercle*, **72**, 1–6

Konno, K. (1956) New chemical method to differentiate human type tubercle bacilli from other mycobacteria. *Science*, **124**, 985

Koukila-Kähkölä, P., Springer, B., Böttger, E. *et al.* (1995) *Mycobacterium branderi* sp. nov., a new potential human pathogen. *International Journal of Systematic Bacteriology*, **45**, 549–553

Kubica, G.P. (1973) Differential identification of mycobacteria IV. Key features for identification of clinically significant mycobacteria. *American Review of Respiratory Disease*, **107**, 9–21

Kubica, G.P. (1980) Correlation of acid-fast staining methods with culture results for mycobacteria. *Bulletin of the International Union Against Tuberculosis*, **55**, 117–124

Kubica, G.P., Silcox, V.A., Kilburn, J.O. *et al.* (1970) Differential identification of mycobacteria. VI. *Mycobacterium triviale* Kubica sp. nov. *International Journal of Systematic Bacteriology*, **20**, 164–174

Kubica, G.P., Baess, I., Gordon, R.E. *et al.* (1972) Numerical analysis of rapidly growing mycobacteria. *Journal of General Microbiology*, **73**, 55–70

Kubica, G.P., Gross, W.M., Hawkins, J.E. *et al.* (1975) Laboratory services for mycobacterial disease. *American Review of Respiratory Disease*, **112**, 773–787

Küster, E. (1905) Über Kaltblutertuberkulose. *Münchener Medizinische Wochenschrift*, **52**, 57–59

Kusunoki, S. and Ezaki, T. (1992) Proposal of *Mycobacterium peregrinum* sp. nov., nom. rev., and elevation of *Mycobacterium chelonae* subsp. *abscessus* (Kubica *et al*) to species *Mycobacterium abscessus* comb. nov. *International Journal of Systematic Bacteriology*, **42**, 240–245

Kvach, J.T., Munguia, G. and Strand, S.H. (1984) Staining tissue-derived *Mycobacterium leprae* with fluorescein diacetate and ethidium bromide. *International Journal of Leprosy*, **52**, 176–182

Leat, J.L. and Marks, J. (1970) Improvement on drug-sensitivity tests on tubercle bacilli. *Tubercle*, **51**, 68–73

Lehmann, K.B. and Neumann, R. (1896) *Atlas und Grundriss der Bakteriologie und Lehrbuch der speciellen bakteriologischen Diagnostik.* 1st edn. Munich: J. F. Lehmann

Lehmann, K.B. and Neumann, R. (1899) *ibid.* 2nd edn. pp. 408–413

Levy-Frebault, V., Rafidinarivo, E., Prome, J.C., *et al.* (1983) *Mycobacterium fallax* sp. nov. *International Journal of Systematic Bacteriology*, **33**, 336–343

Linell, F. and Norden, A. (1954) *Mycobacterium balnei*: a new acid-fast bacillus occurring in swimming pools and capable of producing skin lesions in humans. *Acta Tuberculosea Scandinavica, Supplement.* **33**, 1–84

Luquin, M., Ausina, V., Vincent-Lévy-Frébault, V. *et al.* (1993) *Mycobacterium brumae* sp. nov., a rapidly growing, nonphotochromogenic mycobacterium. *International Journal of Systematic Bacteriology*, **43**, 405–413

MacCallum, P., Tolhurst, J.C., Buckle, G. and Sissons, H.A. (1948) A new mycobacterial infection of man. *Journal of Pathology and Bacteriology*, **60**, 93–122

McFadden, J.J., Van Der Giessen, J.W.B., Haring, R.M. and Van Der Zeijst, B.A.M. (1994) Comparison of the 23S ribosomal RNA genes and the spacer region between the 16S and 23S rRNA genes of the closely related *Mycobacterium avium* and *Mycobacterium paratuberculosis* and the fast-growing *Mycobacterium phlei*. *Journal of General Microbiology*, **140**, 1103–1108

M'Fadyean, J. (1907) Johne's disease: chronic bacterial enteritis of cattle. *Journal of Comparative Pathology and Therapeutics*, **20**, 48–60

Manten, A. (1957) Antimicrobial susceptibility and some other properties of photochromogenic mycobacteria associated with pulmonary disease. *Antonie van Leeuwenhoek*, **23**, 357–363

Marchoux, E. and Sorel, F. (1912) Recherches sur la lepré. *Annales de l'Institut Pasteur*, **26**, 675–700

Marks, J. (1958). Indeterminate mycobacteria. *British Journal of Clinical Practice*, **12**, 763

Marks, J. (1961) The design of sensitivity tests on tubercle bacilli. *Tubercle*, **42**, 314–316

Marks, J. (1964a) A 'stepped pH' technique for the estimation of pyrazinamide sensitivity. *Tubercle*, **45**, 47–50

Marks, J. (1964b) Aspects of epidemiology of infection by 'anonymous' mycobacteria. *Proceedings of the Royal Society of Medicine*, **57**, 479–480

Marks, J. (1972) Classification of mycobacteria in relation to clinical significance. *Tubercle*, **53**, 259–264

Marks, J. (1976) A system for the examination of tubercle bacilli and other mycobacteria. *Tubercle*, **57**, 207–225

Marks, J. and Szulga, T. (1965) Thin layer chromatography of mycobacterial lipids as an aid to classification. Technical procedures: *Mycobacterium fortuitum*. *Tubercle*, **46**, 400–411

Marks, J. and Trollope, D.R. (1960) A study of the anonymous mycobacteria. *Tubercle*, **41**, 51–62

Marks, J., Jenkins, P.A. and Tsukamura, M. (1972) *Mycobacterium szulgai*: a new pathogen. *Tubercle*, **53**, 210–214

Meissner, G. (1964) The bacteriology of the tubercle bacillus. In: *The Chemotherapy of Tuberculosis*. Barry, V.C., ed. London: Butterworths

Meissner, G. and Schroder, K. (1975) Relationship between *Mycobacterium simiae* and *Mycobacterium habana*. *American Review of Respiratory Disease*, **111**, 196

Meyers, W.M. (1995) Mycobacterial infections of the skin. In Seifert, G (ed.) *Tropical Pathology*. Heidelberg: Springer-Verlag. pp. 291–337

Middlebrook, G. and Cohn, M.L. (1958) Bacteriology of tuberculosis: laboratory methods. *American Journal of Public Health*, 48: 844–853

Miller, N., Hernandez, S.G. and Cleary, T.J. (1994) Evaluation of Gen-Probe Amplified Mycobacterium Tuberculosis Direct Test and PCR for direct detection of *Mycobacterium tuberculosis* in clinical specimens. *Journal of Clinical Microbiology*, **32**, 393–397

Mitchison, D.A. (1982) Organisation of tuberculosis laboratory services in developing countries. *Bulletin of the International Union Against Tuberculosis*, **57**, 140–147

Mitchison, D.A., Allen, B.W., Carroll, L., Dickinson, J.M. and Aber, V.R. (1972) A selective oleic acid medium for tubercle bacilli. *Journal of Medical Microbiology*, **5**, 165–175

Mitchison, D.A., Allen, B.W. and Manickavasagar, D. (1983) Selective Kirchner medium in the culture of specimens other than sputum for mycobacteria. *Journal of Clinical Pathology*, **36**, 1357–1361

Moore, M. and Frerichs, J.B. (1953) An unusual acid-fast infection of the knee, with subcutaneous abscess-like lesions in the gluteal region. *Journal of Investigative Dermatology*, **20**, 133–169

Nitta, A.T., Davidson, P.T., De Koning, M.L. *et al.* (1996) Misdiagnosis of multidrug resistant tuberculosis possibly due to laboratory-related errors. *Journal of the American Medical Association*, **276**, 1980–1983

Nordhoek, G.T., Kolk, A.H.J., Bjune, G. *et al.* (1994) Sensitivity and specificity of PCR for detection of *Mycobacterium tuberculosis*: a blind comparison study among seven laboratories, *Journal of Clinical Microbiology*, **32**, 277–284

Ohashi, D.K., Wade, T.J. and Mandle, R.J. (1977) Characterisation of ten species of mycobacteria by reaction-gas-liquid chromatography. *Journal of Clinical Microbiology*, **6**, 469–473

Penso, G., Castelnuova, G., Gaudiano, A. *et al.* (1952) Studi e richerche sui micobatteri VIII. Un bacillo tuberculare: il *Mycobacterium minetti* n.sp. Studio microbiologica e patogenico. *Rendiconti dell' Instituto Superiore di Sanita, Roma*, **15**, 491–548

Portaels, F., Fonteyne, P.-A., De Beenhouwer, H. *et al.* (1996a) Variability in 3′ end of 16S rRNA sequence of *Mycobacterium ulcerans* is related to geographic origin of isolates. *Journal of Clinical Microbiology*, **34**, 962–965

Portaels, F., Realini, L. and Bauwens, L. *et al.* (1996b) Mycobacteriosis caused by *Mycobacterium genavense* in birds kept in a zoo: an 11 year survey. *Journal of Clinical Microbiology*, **34**, 319–323

Prissick, F.H. and Masson, A.M. (1956) Cervical lymphadenitis in children caused by chromogenic mycobacteria. *Canadian Medical Association Journal*, **3**, 91–100

Public Health Laboratory Service (1966) Regional Centres for Tuberculosis Bacteriology. *Monthly Bulletin of the Ministry of Health and the Public Health Laboratory Service*, **25**, 36

Rastogi, N. and Falkinham, J.O. (eds.) (1996) Solving the dilemma of antimycobacterial chemotherapy. *Research in Microbiology*, **147**, 7–121

Reed, G.B. (1957) Family 1 Mycobacteriaceae Chester 1897. In: *Bergey's Manual of Determinative Bacteriology* 7th ed. Eds Breed, R.S., Murray, E.G.D. and Smith, N.R. Baltimore: Williams and Wilkins

Richmond, J.Y. and McKinney, R.W. (eds.) (1993) *Biosafety in microbiological and biomedical laboratories*, 3rd edn. Washington, D.C., U.S. Government Printing Office. Health and Human Services publication (CDC) 93–8395, 1993

Ridley, D.S. (1988) *Pathogenesis of Leprosy and Related Diseases*. London: Wright.

Ridley, D.S. and Jopling W.H. (1966) Classification of leprosy according to immunity: a five-group system. *International Journal of Leprosy*, **34**, 255–273

Rieder, H.L. (1994) Tuberculosis and human immunodeficiency virus infection in industrialized countries. In Davies P.D.O. (ed.) *Clinical Tuberculosis*. London, Chapman and Hall. pp. 227–240

Rist, N., Canetti, G., Boisvert, H. and Le Lirzin, M. (1967) L'antibiogramme du BCG. Valeur diagnostique de la resistance a la cycloserine. *Revue de Tuberculose et de Pneumonologie*, **31**, 1060–1065

Rogall, T., Flohr, T. and Böttger, E.C. (1990) Differentiation of *Mycobacterium* species by direct sequencing of amplified DNA. *Journal of General Microbiology*, **136**, 1915–1920

Rouillon, A., Perdrizet, S. and Parrot, R. (1976) Transmission of tubercle bacilli: the effects of chemotherapy. *Tubercle*, **57**, 275–299

Runyon, E.H. (1959) Anonymous mycobacteria in pulmonary disease. *Medical Clinics of North America*, **43**, 273–290

Runyon, E.H. (1965) Pathogenic mycobacteria. *Advances in Tuberculosis Research*, **14**, 235–287

Runyon, E.H. (1967) *Mycobacterium intracellulare. American Review of Respiratory Disease*, **95**, 861–867

Runyon, E.H. (1972) Conservation of the specific epithet *fortuitum* in the name of the organism known as *Mycobacterium fortuitum* da Costa Cruz. Request for an opinion. *International Journal of Systematic Bacteriology*, **22**, 50–51

Runyon, E.H., Bönicke, R., Buchanan, R.E. *et al.* (1967) *Mycobacterium tuberculosis, M. bovis* and *M. microti* species descriptions. *Zentralblatt für Bakteriologie, Parasitenkunde, Infektionskrankheiten und Hygiene*, Abteilung I Originale, **204**, 405–413

Runyon, E.H., Wayne, L.G. and Kubica, G.P. (1974) Family II Mycobacteriaceae Chester 1897, 63. In: *Bergey's Manual of Determinative Bacteriology* 8th edn. (Buchanan, R.E. and Gibbons, eds.) N.E. Baltimore: Williams and Wilkins

Russell, A.D. (1996) Activity of biocides against mycobacteria. *Journal of Applied Bacteriology* **81**, 87S–101S.

Russell, A.D., Hugo, W.B. and Ayliffe, G.A.J. (1992) *Principles and Practice of Disinfection, Preservation and Sterilization*. Oxford: Blackwell Scientific

Saceanu, C.A., Pfeiffer, N.C., McLean, T. (1993) Evaluation of sputum smears concentrated by cytocentrifugation for detection of acid-fast bacilli. *Journal of Clinical Microbiology*, **31**, 2371–2374

Salfinger, M. and Morris, A.J. (1994) The role of the microbiology laboratory in diagnosing mycobacterial diseases. *American Journal of Clinical Pathology*, **101** Suppl. 1 (Pathology Patterns), S6-S13

Salfinger, M. and Pfyffer, G.E. (1994) The new diagnostic mycobacteriology laboratory. *European Journal of Clinical Mycobacteriology and Infectious Diseases*, **13**, 961–979

Salfinger, M., Demchik, B.S. and Kafader, F.M. (1990) Comparison between the MB Check system, radiometric and conventional methods for recovery of mycobacteria. *Journal of Microbiological Methods*, **12**, 97–100

Schaefer, W.B. (1965) Serological identification and classification of the atypical mycobacteria by their agglutination. *American Review of Respiratory Disease*, **92**, Supplement, 85–93

Schröder, K.H. and Juhlin, I. (1977) *Mycobacterium malmoense* sp. nov. *International Journal of Systematic Bacteriology*, **27**, 241–246

Schwabacher, H. (1959) A strain of mycobacterium isolated from skin lesions of a cold-blooded animal *Xenopus laevis*, and its relation to atypical acid-fast bacilli occurring in man. *Journal of Hygiene*, **57**, 57–67

Shaw, R. (1994) Polymerase chain reaction. In *Clinical Tuberculosis*. (Davies, PDO, ed.) London: Chapman and Hall. pp. 381–389

Sims, B. (1991) Laboratory waste, our "duty of care". *IMLS Gazette*, August 1991, pp. 416–420

Skerman, V.D.B., McGowan, V. and Sneath, P.H.A. (1980) Approved lists of bacterial names. *International Journal of Systematic Bacteriology*, **30**, 225–420

Slutsky, A.M., Arbeit, R.D., Barber, T.W. *et al.* (1994) Polyclonal infections due to *Mycobacterium avium* complex in patients with AIDS detected by pulsed field gel electrophoresis of sequential clinical isolates. *Journal of Clinical Microbiology*, **32**, 1173–1178

Smith, T. (1898) A comparative study of bovine tubercle bacilli and of human bacilli from sputum. *Journal of Experimental Medicine*, **3**, 451–551

Sommers, H.M. and McClatchy, J.K. (1983) *Laboratory Diagnosis of the Mycobacterioses* (CUMI-TECH 16). Washington: The American Society for Microbiology

Sompolinsky, D., Lagziel, A., Naveh, D. and Yankilevitz, T. (1978) *Mycobacterium haemophilum* sp. nov. A new pathogen of humans. *International Journal of Systematic Bacteriology*, **28**, 67–75

Spigelman, M. and Lemma, E. (1993) The use of the polymerase chain reaction (PCR) to detect *Mycobacterium tuberculosis* in ancient skeletons. *International Journal of Osteoarchaeology*, **3**, 137–143

Standards Association of Australia (1983) *AS 2647: Biological Safety Cabinets – Installation and Use*. Sydney: SAA

Stanford, J.L. and Grange, J.M. (1974) The meaning and structure of species as applied to mycobacteria. *Tubercle*, **55**, 143–152

Stanford, J.L. and Gunthorpe, W.J. (1969) Serological and bacteriological investigation of *Mycobacterium ranae* (*fortuitum*). *Journal of Bacteriology*, **98**, 375–383

Stanford, J.L. and Gunthorpe, W.J. (1971) A study of some fast-growing scotochromogens including species descriptions of *Mycobacterium gilvum* (new species) and *Mycobacterium duvalii* (new species). *British Journal of Experimental Pathology*, **52**, 627–637

Stoker, N. (1994) Tuberculosis in a changing world. *British Medical Journal*, **309**, 1178–1179

Suzanne, M. and Penso, G. (1953) Sulla identita specifiea de cosidetto 'ceppo Chauvire' *Mycobacterium marianum* nov. sp. *Riuassunto delle Communicazione del VI Congresso Internazionale de Microbiologia (Roma)*, **2**, 655–656

Taik Chae Kim, Blackman, R.S., Heatwole, K.M. *et al.* (1984) Acid-fast bacilli in sputum smears of patients with pulmonary tuberculosis. *American Review of Respiratory Disease*, **129**, 264–268

Tan Thiam Hok (1962) A simple and rapid cold staining method for acid-fast bacteria. *American Review of Respiratory Disease*, **85**, 753–754

Telenti, A., Imboden, P., Marchesi, F. *et al.* (1993) Direct automated detection of rifampin-resistant *Mycobacterium tuberculosis* by polymerase chain reaction and single strand conformation polymorphism analysis. *Antimicrobial Agents and Chemotherapy*, **37**, 2054–2058

Telles, M.A.S. and Yates, M.D. (1994) Single and double drug susceptibility testing of *Mycobacterium avium* complex and other MOTT bacilli by a microdilution broth MIC method. *Tubercle and Lung Disease*, **75**, 286–290

Timpe, A. and Runyon, E.H. (1954) The relationship of 'atypical' acid-fast bacteria to human disease: a preliminary report. *Journal of Laboratory and Clinical Medicine*, **44**, 202–209

Tisdall, P.A., DeYoung, D.R., Roberts, G.D. and Anhalt, J.P. (1982) Identification of clinical isolates of mycobacteria with gas-liquid chromatography: a 10-month follow-up study. *Journal of Clinical Microbiology*, **16**, 400–402

Tisdall, P.A., Roberts, G.D. and Anhalt, I.P. (1979) Identification of clinical isolates of mycobacteria with gas-liquid chromatography alone. *Journal of Clinical Microbiology*, **10**, 506–514

Tomioka, H., Saito, H. and Sato, K. (1992) *Mycobacterium leprae* activity of various antimicrobials. *Japanese Journal of Leprosy*, **61**, 157–164

Tsukamura, M. (1965) A group of mycobacteria from soil sources resembling nonphotochromogens (Group III). A description of *Mycobacterium nonchromogenicum*. *Medicine and Biology*, **71**, 110–113

Tsukamura, M. (1966a) *Mycobacterium parafortuitum*: a new species. *Journal of General Microbiology*, **42**, 7–12

Tsukamura, M. (1966b) Adansonian classification of mycobacteria. *Journal of General Microbiology*, **45**, 253–273

Tsukamura, M. (1966c) *Mycobacterium chitae*, a new species. Preliminary report. *Medicine and Biology*, **73**, 203–205

Tsukamura, M. (1967) Two types of slowly growing, nonphotochromogenic mycobacteria obtained from soil by the mouse passage method. *Mycobacterium terrae* and *Mycobacterium novum*. *Japanese Journal of Microbiology*, **11**, 163–172

Tsukamura, M. (1970) Screening for atypical mycobacteria. *Tubercle*, **51**, 280–284

Tsukamura, M. (1972) A new species of rapidly growing, scotochromogenic mycobacteria, *Mycobacterium neoaurum* Tsukamura n. sp. *Medicine and Biology*, **85**, 229–233

Tsukamura, M. (1974) Niacin negative *Mycobacterium tuberculosis*. *American Review of Respiratory Disease*, **110**, 101–103

Tsukamura, M. (1981) Numerical analysis of rapidly growing nonphotochromogenic mycobacteria, including *Mycobacterium agri* sp. nov., nom. rev. *International Journal of Systematic Bacteriology*, **31**, 247–258

Tsukamura, M. (1982) *Mycobacterium shimoidei* sp. nov., nom. rev. A lung pathogen. *International Journal of Systematic Bacteriology*, **32**, 67–69

Tsukamura, M. and Tsukamura, S. (1964) Differentiation of *Mycobacterium tuberculosis* and *Mycobacterium bovis* by *p*-nitrobenzoic acid susceptibility. *Tubercle*, **45**, 64–65

Tsukamura, M., Mizuno, S., Gane, N.F.F. *et al.* (1971) *Mycobacterium rhodesiae* sp. nov. A new species of rapidly growing sotochromogenic mycobacteria. *Japanese Journal of Microbiology*, **15**, 407–416

Tsukamura, M., Van Der Meulen, H.J. and Grabow, W.O.K. (1983a) Numerical analysis of rapidly growing scotochromogenic mycobacteria of the *Mycobacterium parafortuitum* complex: *Mycobacterium austroafricanum* sp. nov. and *Mycobacterium diernhoferi* sp. nov., nom. rev. *International Journal of Systematic Bacteriology*, **33**, 460–469

Tsukamura, M., Nemoto, T. and Yugi, H. (1983b) *Mycobacterium porcium* sp. nov., a porcine pathogen. *International Journal of Systematic Bacteriology*, **33**, 162–165

Tsukamura, M., Mizuno, S. and Toyama, H. (1983c) *Mycobacterium pulveris* sp. nov., a nonphotochromogenic mycobacterium with an intermediate growth rate. *International Journal of Systematic Bacteriology*, **33**, 811–815

Tsukamura, M., Yano, I. and Imaeda, T. (1986) *Mycobacterium moriokaense* sp. nov., A rapidly growing nonphotochromogenic *Mycobacterium*. *International Journal of Systematic Bacteriology*, **36**, 333–338

Tsukamura, M., Kaneda, K., Imaeda, T. and Mikoshiba, H. (1989) A taxonomic study on a *Mycobacterium* which caused skin ulcer in a Japanese girl and resembled *Mycobacterium ulcerans*. *Kekkaku*, **64**, 691–697

Valdivia-Alvarez, J., Suarez-Mendez, R. and Echemendia-Font, M. (1971) *Mycobacterium habana*: probable nueva especie dentro de la micobatterias. *Boletin de Higiene Epidemiologia*, **8**, 65–73

Van Embden, J.D.A., Cave, M.D. and Crawford, J.T. (1993) Strain identification of *Mycobacterium tuberculosis* by DNA fingerprinting: recommendations for a standardised methodology. *Journal of Clinical Microbiology*, **31**, 406–409

Van Soolingen, D., De Haas, P.E.W., Haagsma, J. *et al.* (1994) Use of various genetic markers in differentiation of *Mycobacterium bovis* strains from animals and humans and for studying epidemiology of bovine tuberculosis. *Journal of Clinical Microbiology*, **32**, 2425–2433

Vestal, A.L. (1975) *Procedures for the Isolation and Identification of Mycobacteria*. DHEW Publication no. (CDC) 75-8230. Atlanta: Centers for Disease Control

Vincke, G., Yegers, O., Vanachter, H. *et al.* (1982) Rapid susceptibility testing of *Mycobacterium tuberculosis* by a radiometric technique. *Journal of Antimicrobial Chemotherapy*, **10**, 351–354

Vuorinen, P., Miettinen, A., Vuento, R. and Hällström, O. (1995) Direct detection of *Mycobacterium tuberculosis* complex in respiratory specimens by Gen-Probe Mycobacterium Tuberculosis Direct Test and Roche Amplicor Mycobacterium Tuberculosis Test. *Journal of Clinical Microbiology*, **33**, 1856–1859

Wallace, R.J., Zhang, Y., Brown, B.A. *et al.* (1993) DNA large restriction fragment patterns of sporadic and epidemic nosocomial strains of *Mycobacterium chelonae* and *Mycobacterium abscessus*. *Journal of Clinical Microbiology*, **31**, 2697–2701

Wallgren, A. (1948) The timetable of tuberculosis. *Tubercle*, **29**, 245–251

Wayne, L.G. (1964) Nomenclature of the mycobacteria. *American Review of Respiratory Disease*, **90**, 278

Wayne, L.G. (1966) Classification and identification of mycobacteria III. Species within Group III. *American Review of Respiratory Disease*, **93**, 919–928

Wayne, L.G. (1968) *Mycobacterium marinum* and *Mycobacterium marianum*. *American Review of Respiratory Disease*, **98**, 317

Wayne, L.G. (1970) On the identity of *Mycobacterium gordonae* Bojalil and the so-called tap water scotochromogens. *International Journal of Systematic Bacteriology*, **20**, 149–153

Wayne, L.G. (1975) Proposal to reject the specific epithet marianum in the name *Mycobacterium marianum* Penso 1953 and to conserve the specific epithet in the name *Mycobacterium scrofulaceum* Prissick and Masson 1956. Request for an opinion. *International Journal of Systematic Bacteriology*, **25**, 230–231

Wayne, L.G. (1979) Simple pyrazinamidase and urease tests for routine identification of mycobacteria. *American Review of Respiratory Disease*, **109**, 147–151

Wayne, L.G. and Krasnow, I. (1966) Preparation of tuberculosis sensitivity medium by means of impregnated discs. *American Journal of Clinical Pathology*, **45**, 769–771

Weiszfeiler, J.G., Karasseva, V. and Karczag, E. (1971) A new *Mycobacterium* species: *Mycobacterium asiaticum* n. sp. *Acta Microbiologica Academiae Scientarum Hungarica*, **18**, 247–252

Weiten, G., Haverkamp, J., Meuzelaar, H.L.C., Engel, H.W.B. and Berwald, L.G. (1981) Pyrolysis mass spectrometry: a new method to differentiate between the mycobacteria of the 'tuberculosis complex' and other mycobacteria. *Journal of General Microbiology*, **122**, 109–118

Wells A.Q. (1946) *The Murine Type of Tubercle Bacillus*. Medical Research Council Special Report no. 259 London: HMSO

Williams, D.L., Waguespack, C., Eisenach, K. *et al.* (1994) Characterization of rifampin resistance in pathogenic mycobacteria. *Antimicrobial Agents and Chemotherapy*, **38**, 2380–2386

Wilson, S.M., McNerney, R., Nye, P.M. *et al.* (1993) Progress towards a simplified polymerase chain reaction and its application to the diagnosis of tuberculosis. *Journal of Clinical Microbiology* **31**, 776–782

Wolinsky, E. (1979) Non-tuberculous mycobacteria and associated diseases. *American Review of Respiratory Disease*, **119**, 107–159

Woods, G.L. and Witebsky, F.G. (1995) Mycobacterial testing in clinical laboratories that participate in the College of American Pathologists' mycobacteriology E survey: results of a 1993 questionnaire. *Journal of Clinical Microbiology*, **33**, 407–412

World Health Organization (1993a) *Laboratory Biosafety Manual*, 2nd edn. Geneva: WHO

World Health Organization (1993b) *Treatment of tuberculosis. Guidelines for national programmes.* Geneva: WHO

World Health Organization (1994) *Chemotherapy of leprosy.* Technical Report Series No. 847. Geneva: WHO

World Health Organization (1995) *Stop TB at the source. WHO report on the tuberculosis epidemic, 1995.* Geneva: WHO publication WHO/TB/95.183

Yano, K., Kagayama, K., Ohmo, Y. *et al.* (1978) Separation and analysis of molecular species of mycolic acids in *Nocardia* and related taxa by gas chromatography mass spectrometry. *Biomedical Mass Spectrometry*, **5**, 14–24

Yates, M.D. (1984) The differentiation and epidemiology of the tubercle bacilli and a study into the identification of other mycobacteria. MPhil Thesis: University of London

Yates, M.D. and Collins, C.H. (1979) Identification of tubercle bacilli. *Annales de Microbiologie*, **130B**, 13–19

Yates, M.D., Collins, C.H. and Grange, J.M. (1978) Differentiation of BCG from other variants of *Mycobacterium tuberculosis* isolated from clinical material. *Tubercle*, **59**, 143–146

Yates, M.D., Grange, J.M. and Collins, C.H. (1984) A study of the relationship between the resistance of *Mycobacterium tuberculosis* to isonicotinic acid hydrazide (isoniazid) and to thiophen-2-carboxylic acid hydrazide. *Tubercle*, **65**, 295–299

Zaher, F. and Marks, J. (1977) Methods and medium for the culture of tubercle bacilli. *Tubercle*, **58**, 143–145

Zhang, Y., Mazurek, G.H., Cave, M.D. *et al.* (1992) DNA polymorphisms in strains of *Mycobacterium tuberculosis* analyzed by pulsed-field gel electrophoresis: a tool for epidemiology. *Journal of Clinical Microbiology*, **30**, 1551–1556

Appendix

Assay of antimicrobial agents in serum and their detection in urine

It is only rarely necessary to determine serum levels of antimycobacterial agents. The first line antituberculosis drugs, isoniazid, rifampicin and pyrazinamide (and also ethionamide), are destroyed by metabolism or excreted in the bile. They may therefore be used safely in patients with renal failure. Streptomycin and ethambutol, on the other hand, are almost entirely eliminated by the kidneys. There are several rapid assays for streptomycin: these include high pressure liquid chromatography and enzyme immunoassays. Standard microbial assays are, however, usually adequate although it is important to use a test organism that is resistant to all other antibacterial agents that the patient is receiving. For details of these assays see Collins *et al*. (1995). An accumulation of ethambutol can lead to the serious complication of optic neuritis. Unfortunately, the assay of this agent is a complex one that is not readily available. Ethambutol is therefore best avoided in cases of renal impairment.

The rate of elimination of isoniazid from the body depends on the rapidity of its acetylation in the liver. This metabolic activity is genetically controlled and the population is divisible into slow and rapid acetylators. This, however, does not affect the therapeutic efficacy of isoniazid if given daily, thrice weekly or twice weekly. The half-life is only increased by up to 30% in almost complete renal failure, even in slow acetylators. There is therefore is no need to determine either the acetylator status of the patients or their serum isoniazid levels.

'Spot tests' for antituberculosis or antileprosy drugs or their metabolites in urine have been used to check patient compliance although such tests are no substitute for well-organized directly observed therapy.

Urine test for isoniazid

This is best undertaken with commercially available test strips (Difco). The urine is positive for 24 hours or more after ingestion of 100 mg of isoniazid. (The more formal method requires use of potentially dangerous chemicals, potassium cyanide and barbituric acid, and is thus best avoided.)

Urine test for rifampicin

This test is based on the red colour of rifampicin and its metabolite desacetyl-rifampicin. Add 2 ml of N-butanol to 10 ml of urine and mix gently by inverting the tube twice. Place the tube upright to allow the butanol to form a separate upper layer. The presence of the drug is indicated by a pink or red coloration of this layer. An excess of bile in the urine can cause a similar coloration.

Urine test for dapsone

Place one drop of fresh urine on a strip of filter paper impregnated with Ehrlich's reagent (p-dimethylaminobenzaldehyde, 1 g; N hydrochloric acid, 20 ml; ethanol, 80 ml). A central orange coloured spot indicates the presence of dapsone. Ignore a yellow ring at the periphery: this is caused by urea. Include dapsone-free urine as a control.

Index